THE CARNIVORE DIET BIBLE

STEPHEN BAKER

© *Copyright 2019 - All rights reserved.*

Legal Notice:

This book is copyright protected. This book is only for personal use. You cannot amend, distribute, sell, use, quote or paraphrase any part, or the content within this book, without the consent of the author or publisher.

Disclaimer Notice:

Please note the information contained within this document is for educational and entertainment purposes only. All effort has been executed to present accurate, up to date, and reliable, complete information. No warranties of any kind are declared or implied. Readers acknowledge that the author is not engaging in the rendering of legal, financial, medical or professional advice.

This book is not intended to be a substitute for the medical advice of a licensed physician. The reader should consult with their doctor in any matters relating to his/her health.

Contents

Introduction 1
History Of The Carnivore Diet 5
Health Benefits You Can Expect 11
Even More Health Benefits! 19
The Carnivore Diet In Detail 29
Do Not Fear Fat 33
Foods To Avoid 39
What To Drink 47
How To Start The Diet 56
Making A Meal Plan 73
Supercharge Your Results 78
Are There Any Downsides? 84
Who Should Avoid The Diet? 90
Walk On The Wild Side 92
Advice On Eating Out 100
Frequently Asked Questions 104
Conclusion 110
30 Easy Carnivore Recipes 112

    Classic Roast Chicken 114

    Eggs and Bacon 116

    Simple Salmon 118

    Oven-Baked Pork Ribs 120

    Pulled Chicken 122

    Meat Cupcakes 125

    Traditional Cod 127

Grill-Smoked Ribs	129
Omelet and Bacon	131
Pulled Beef	133
Meat Pizza	135
Grilled Chicken Wings	138
Lamb Chops	140
Pulled Pork	143
Bacon Burgers	145
Fried Liver	147
Fresh Oysters	149
Bacon-Crusted Chicken	151
Homemade Jerky	153
Pork Sausages	155
Simple Turkey Breast	157
Carnivore Cheese Balls	160
Pork Belly	162
Classic Steak	164
Chicken Liver Pâté	166
Grilled Shrimp	168
Poached Rainbow Trout	170
Carnivore Steak Nuggets	172
Beginner's Bone Broth	174
Duck Leg Confit	176
Further Resources	178
About the Author	180

For my wife, Andrea, and children, Emma and Jacob. You are the reason why I want to live a long and healthy life.

Introduction

Congratulations on purchasing the *Carnivore Diet Bible* and taking the first step to a new healthy lifestyle. You have probably heard the old adage *"you are what you eat,"* but as our knowledge of the human body grows day by day, this saying rings truer than ever. What we put inside our bodies is vital to our overall health — more so than any other factor. This is especially true in our modern age, when the composition of food has seen drastic changes over the past century — and not for the better.

How we nourish our bodies is not only the key to better health but also to a better quality of life. A nutritionally poor diet will leave us low on energy, fatigued and robs us of the chance to become all we can be. Conversely, a diet full of good nutritious choices, which includes all the essential vitamins and minerals we need, will give us clean energy that will not pollute our systems and leave us lagging behind in life.

As science grows to understand the fundamentals of health more and more, we cannot underestimate the importance of the link between diet choices and health outcomes. As a result, we now appreciate that at the very heart of anything we want to achieve in our lives, good nutrition is essential. No matter what your dreams are, if your body is not nutritionally balanced, with the right amount of minerals, proteins and vitamins, you will struggle to attain success in any field.

For years, many so-called health experts have been advocating a switch to a 100 per cent plant-based diet, either as a vegetarian or a vegan. If this was a natural form of eating, you would think that it would be easy for people to accept and incorporate this kind of change in their eating habits. However, in a world of almost 8 billion people, it is estimated that, as of the end of 2018, there were only 1.5 billion who are vegetarians, and of that number only 75 million are vegetarians by choice. The others are doing so mainly for religious, family or societal reasons. It seems people innately know that meat in the diet is good for them.

These statistics show that regardless of what people are saying about the dangers of meat (especially red meat), something inside of us as a species just does not want to let it go. This is one of the main reasons why the carnivore diet is gaining in popularity. It is connecting us back to our traditional evolutionary roots and, in most cases, was the only diet our ancestors knew and thrived on.

So the carnivore diet is not new. It has been around for thousands upon thousands of years, but here in the following pages the information you will learn might be new to you — or it may be something you have already instinctively understood. Regardless, this book is designed as a one-stop resource for everything you will ever need to know concerning the carnivore diet, including how to use it to your advantage for optimum health, a muscular and athletic body, and fast fat loss.

The following chapters will discuss what the carnivore diet is and how it rose to popularity. We will go into detail about the results you can expect from the diet and the host of benefits that you will love. We will include the obstacles you may need to overcome and provide a detailed do's-and-don'ts guide to mastering this unique diet. Plus, to top it all off, we have thirty delicious recipes that are easy on the wallet, easy on the stomach and approved for the carnivore diet.

Thanks again for choosing the Carnivore Diet Bible. Every effort was made to ensure it is packed full of useful information. Read, enjoy, take notes and then implement — as that is when the magic happens.

Stephen Baker

History Of The Carnivore Diet

To begin our dive into the carnivore diet let's look at what the term "carnivore" really means, as that can give you a pretty clear idea of what the diet itself will entail. "Carnivore" is a Latin-based word that roughly translates to "meat eater", which is why we use it today as a label for animals that can only survive off protein such as big cats or birds of prey.

While advocates for plant-based diets will push their views based on environmental conditions, empathy for fellow creatures, or for some other societal issue, the one fact they often ignore is that meat has been crucial to mankind's survival and evolution. A simple look at the history of our species is evidence of this fact.

For millennia our diet did not change much. In fact, at one time, most societies had diets that consisted almost entirely of meat and little else. During those times, diseases that are all-too-common today did not exist. Diabetes, heart disease, cancer and an entire host of autoimmune diseases that are running rampant in our modern society were not in evidence.

Of course, as archaeologists and anthropologists paw through centuries of historical data, it is not likely that they have come across a three-million-year-old cookbook. However, by examining the remains and artifacts of our distant ancestors, along with the implements and tools they used, we know that the primary part of their diet consisted of meat.

At this point, you might be wondering why you should care what was eaten three million years ago or even five hundred years ago for that matter. It is important because we pretty much have the same DNA and body composition as our ancestors. If their bodies were more accustomed to meat than plants, it is undeniable that we still have the same mechanisms at work in us today. History tells us that meat was the fuel that allowed the human race to not only survive, but to grow in stature and evolve in brain power.

Meat was essential for our ancestors' diet because it was an important way to get enough calories into each meal. They did not have a regular three-meals-a-day schedule and had no idea when or where their next meal was coming from. Meat gave them a calorie-dense food source that provided the store of energy they needed to be strong enough for the next hunt.

It was not until we arrived in the agricultural era that our diet began to shift to include more plant-based matter. Agriculture made it possible to have a steadier and more reliable source of food, and it was only at this point that eating regular meals became the norm.

As a result of the first agricultural revolution approximately ten thousand years ago, human diets began to include more and more plant-based foods. In the beginning, the number of grains we ate were minimal. This was due to the fact that technology had not yet been invented that would allow these plant-based foods to be transported to our tables with any regularity. However, since the 1700s, there has been a gradual but steady increase in plant-based foods featuring in our diets. A good part of this new consumption is in the form of carbohydrates and sugars.

In the 1700s, the average person consumed around 4 pounds of sugar a year. In the 1800s, this number had increased to around 22 pounds per person. Today, our consumption of sugar has increased to somewhere in the region of 180 pounds of sugar per person every year. That is simply staggering.

To be clear, this does not mean that we are all eating bags of Snickers bars or apple pies. While those foods are obviously heavily laden with sugar, most of the sugars we consume today are in forms that we are not even aware of. According to the American Heart Association, the average American consumes about 22 teaspoons of sugar every day.

A lot of these sugars are hidden in the foods we have been told are good for our health. As you read labels that say things like "whole grains", "heart healthy" and "no added sugar", you can be forgiven for believing you are feeding yourself and your family nutritious fare. But manufacturers have learnt to disguise the ingredients using names you may not be familiar with. There are at least 60 names for sugar that are allowed to be used on foods labels.

You might easily recognize terms such as glucose or fructose and know what they are, but you may not be familiar with sugars with names like Florida crystals, Muscovado, Panela, Sorghum, Turbinado, Barley Malt, Dextrin, Dextrose,

Diastatic Malt, Maltodextrin, Maltose, Galactose, and so on and so on. When you read food labels you tend to see the big print at the front touting the supposed health benefits, while your eyes simply miss words like these in tiny letters at the back. The end result? You find yourself consuming far more sugar than you ever intended to, or were even aware of.

All this sugar in our diets is in addition to the foods that already contain a good deal of natural sugars, such as fruit. Nor does it include any foods that quickly convert into sugar in your digestive system, such as white rice and pasta. It is almost a guarantee that any processed foods you eat will contain some form of added sugar. The reality is that sugar seems to be in almost everything we eat. Whether we realize it or not, this sugar overload is one of the biggest culprits in keeping us fat, lazy, sluggish and sick. Medical science has shown it is an important contributor to the development of diabetes, cancer and even dementia.

Yet cutting sugar out of our diets is easier said than done. It seems if we do that, there will not be much left on our plate — except for meat, which bring us full circle back to the original diet that our ancestors ate (and thrived on).

Now let's get down to the meat (excuse the pun) of why the carnivore diet is so beneficial.

Health Benefits You Can Expect

There are many reasons why humans naturally want to eat meat. Not only is it flavorful, but we get a sense of satisfaction from meat that we do not get when we consume other food. The texture it offers cannot be mimicked when we consume vegetables and fruits. While they both are chewable food, meat clearly gives our jaws a workout when we eat it. But there are plenty of other reasons why we would instinctively want to reach for that last drumstick across the table.

Protein Power

We often reach for meat because of its great taste and ability to satisfy our hunger, but we also reach for it because we need it at a cellular level. Nutritionally, meat is extremely high in protein. In fact, it is often referred to as a "complete" food source because within it are all the essential amino acids the body needs for health. When you consume an adequate supply of animal proteins, you will not need to take any additional dietary supplements in order to get what you need. You cannot say that of any other food group.

Our bodies are made up of about 20 percent protein. Since the human body is not capable of storing protein, our diets have to be rich in it. We need to find food sources that provide enough protein to sustain us every day.

The human body needs about twenty different amino acids, which can be used to build proteins. These are classified into either essential or non-essential amino acids. The body is capable of producing the non-essential amino acids on its own, but those that are essential can only be acquired through the foods you eat. In addition, they must be acquired in the right ratios so too much of one or too little can counteract the effects of the others.

Animal sources of protein like fish, eggs, poultry and meat are much more closely aligned with the protein your body needs. They contain all the essential ingredients in the right ratios so that your body gets everything it needs to properly function.

Plant proteins, while plentiful, are not as effective in giving the body proper nourishment. They usually will provide some amino acids but are lacking in others. So you may be able to get a plentiful dose of protein from foods such as beans, lentils and nuts, but you will still need to search for other plant sources in order to get the complete complement of proteins your body needs. That is why vegetarians and vegans so often have to take supplements.

To add to that, animal proteins are rarely found by themselves. Meat usually comes with a host of other nutrients essential for human life. So in addition to the critical amino acids, you will also find the following:

- Vitamin B12: from fish, poultry, meat and dairy.
- Vitamin D: from eggs, dairy and oily fish.
- DHA (Docosahexaenoic Acid): an omega-3 fatty acid found in fish.
- Heme-Iron: found mostly in red meat. This form of iron is absorbed by the body more easily than the iron found in plant-based foods. It is very effective in preventing anemia, which can weaken the body.
- Zinc: from beef, pork and lamb.

The bottom line is that meat contains superior forms of protein and essential nutrients which the body needs to survive and thrive.

These nutrients also contribute significantly to better muscle strength and enhance your ability to maintain it as you age. A regular course of meat helps to prevent muscle loss as you get older so that you can maintain your level of endurance and activity for far longer than you could otherwise. It also contributes to better bone strength.

Diets that contain a large proportion of meat have ample amounts of calcium, vitamin D, vitamin B-12 and omega-3 fatty acids, all of which contribute significantly to overall bone health. In addition, B12 promotes better brain development in children and greases the wheels of the neural system so that the brain functions better.

Some may argue that you can get the same nutrients from plants, but there is an important difference. When you consume a primarily plant-based diet, in order to get an adequate supply of all these nutrients, you will need to take vitamin supplements, which are synthetically made.

These synthetic vitamins do not equate to the quality of natural nutrients you get from eating meat, nor does the body absorb them as completely as natural food.

Better Weight Management

One of the most common reasons why people choose the carnivore diet has to do with managing their weight. If you go online and search for "diets and weight loss" you will find an endless stream of contradictory opinions on the best way to do it. One diet that is gaining a lot of traction in this area is the ketogenic diet. Very similar to the carnivore diet, it works for weight loss by restricting the amount of carbohydrates a person consumes, forcing the body into a state of "ketosis".

In ketosis, the body is producing "ketones", which force it to burn fat instead of glucose for its energy, thus the weight loss. The carnivore diet works on that same premise only it is stricter in terms of which foods are allowed. The ketogenic diet allows for some carbohydrates on the menu, but the carnivore diet insists on zero carbs.

Several studies have been conducted that looked closely at how the low-fat restricted-calorie diet, the Mediterranean restricted-calorie diet, and the low-carb non-restricted calorie diet performed. The results were amazing. In 95.4 percent of the participants in these studies, after two years, it was the low-carb non-restricted calorie diet that yielded the best results.

There is a lot of speculation as to why this works. One theory is that while you can eat more calories (non-restrictive), meat tends to be more satiating and therefore you naturally eat less. Basically, you feel full quicker so you consume fewer calories, which will contribute to better weight management. In addition, you have more clean energy so you will burn more calories as well.

There is no question from a scientific point of view that there are many benefits to eliminating carbohydrates and sugars from our diets. Even the natural ones. The health benefits are many. Not only do you get the essential proteins needed for your body to function properly, but you also eliminate exposure to many risk factors that are inherent in the heavy consumption of grains and sugar.

Without the added sugars, your blood glucose levels will be more stable, you lower your chances of developing many autoimmune disorders that can cause painful inflammation throughout the body, and you give your body a huge boost of energy at the same time. Any diet that is 100 percent animal-based is automatically going to give you more fat, which will be much more satisfying and satiating than a plant-based menu. This improves appetite control.

No one really enjoys having to go on a diet. It just seems to be counter-productive to what feels natural. For millennia, humans never had to stop and think about their nutritional needs: they never had to count calories and measure food portions. The way they ate was completely natural and instinctual.

It can be exhausting and discouraging to think about all the little details when following a particular diet regime. That is why so many people are looking for an approach that is simple and easy to follow. When you are on the carnivore diet, you do not have a myriad of factors to worry about, and you can still give your body everything it needs in practically every bite. In fact, it is the kind of diet that, with a little discipline, can easily become a lifestyle because it is so naturally in tune with what our bodies want and need. This makes adherence much easier — and the diet you can stick to is the diet that works!

Even More Health Benefits!

Eating meat is far more satisfying than you might imagine. Due to its high fat content and density, your body will take longer to digest it than any other food group. When you eat carbohydrates, your body quickly uses them up, leaving you empty and hungry and craving something else to eat soon afterwards. The proteins found in meat have to go through a number of hurdles in your digestive system before they can be of use to you. This means they take longer to break down, extending the time when you become hungry again.

Other key benefits of the carnivore diet include:

It Feeds Your Neurotransmitters

Our brains have billions (yes, billions) of neurotransmitters, which are used to experience all of our thoughts, memories and emotions. When they are out of balance, we can suffer from a wide variety of problems, including depression and anxiety disorders. When you have meat as the mainstay of your diet, however, it contributes to keeping your neurotransmitters in balance and healthy, which results in elevated mood and improved cognitive function.

According to one study in the International Journal of Behavioral Nutrition and Physical Activity, people who eat meat fewer than three times a week (and also do not exercise regularly) are more likely to experience mentally stressful conditions such as anxiety and depression. While scientists do not thoroughly understand the mechanism behind this finding, it is believed that the low-level meat eaters are not producing sufficient dopamine, the hormone that gives you a sense of pleasure and well-being. Nor are they receiving an adequate supply of serotonin, which gives you a soothing and peaceful sensation. Both of these hormones are made from amino acids (tyrosine and tryptophan), which are plentiful in meats.

Another study published in the Journal of Affective Disorders revealed that meat eaters are 18 percent less likely to suffer from depression than their vegetarian or vegan counterparts. So the carnivore diet is a sound option for both body and mind.

Allergy Control

An allergic reaction occurs when your immune system determines that a substance in your body represents a threat and action must be taken to get rid of it. It does this by producing antibodies that aim to eliminate the offending allergen. The symptoms you experience can include inflammation of the airwaves, hives, wheezing, chest tightness, shortness of breath or swollen lips, tongue or face.

Many people experience relief when they adopt a more restrictive diet that cuts out foods such as dairy or gluten. However, in modern times we are seeing a sharp increase in allergies due to the consumption of processed foods. These are often loaded toxins, chemicals, preservatives and various forms of sugar that the human body was not designed to ingest.

With the carnivore diet you are nourishing your body with natural foods that have not been chemically altered, genetically modified or exposed to the cornucopia of additives that you find in mass-produced processed food. Your body will not be flooded with a wave of toxins that the immune system then has to fight off.

What is more, there is evidence that fish, which is high in omega-3 fatty acids, can reduce the chances of developing an allergy in the first place. According to the American College of Allergy, Asthma & Immunology, tuna and mackerel are particularly effective at fighting allergies by controlling underlying inflammation, dilating air passages and providing other relief effects from allergens.

Autoimmune Diseases

Similar to allergies, autoimmune diseases result from the immune system becoming overactive and causing the body to attack itself.

Common autoimmune disorders include:

- Rheumatoid arthritis — the immune system attacks the lining of the joints.
- Systemic lupus — the body attacks tissues throughout the body, including the joints, lungs, blood cells, nerves, skin, heart and kidneys.

- IBD (Inflammatory Bowel Disease) — the lining of the intestines is attacked.
- Multiple sclerosis — an attack on the nerve cells leading to pain, vision problems, weakness, muscle spasms and ultimately disability.
- Type 1 Diabetes Mellitus — an attack on insulin-producing cells in the pancreas.

Traditional medicine has made little progress in curing autoimmune diseases and many, such as multiple sclerosis, are still poorly understood. The best modern medicine can do is relieve symptoms.

One theory gaining traction is that autoimmune disorders are the result of ingesting chemically treated plants that are throwing the immune system out of balance (Autoimmune Diseases Journal, February 2014). We are often told that if you eat lots of plants you will be healthier. However, the plants you consume today are not in their natural form. They have been genetically modified, doused with chemical pesticides and grown in environments that are heavily polluted, resulting in a variety of toxins.

Also, like all other living things, plants do not want to be eaten and they have their own internal defense mechanisms. They produce toxins to protect themselves from fungi, insects and animal predators. There are thousands of these natural pesticides and every species of plant has its own set. Like animals (and humans), plants get stressed. When they feel under threat, they increase their production of natural pesticides, which can be detrimental to humans when consumed. These chemicals attack predators in various ways. Some break into cells and kill mitochondria (power generators of cells), some use enzymes to interfere with metabolism, and some attack the DNA directly.

Make no mistake, plants have a dark side, which could well be at the base of a range of modern health problems.

Cardiovascular Health

One of the primary reasons health organizations suggest a limit on the amount of meat you consume is to lower the risk of developing cardiovascular disease. They point out that animal products, in general, contain large amounts of saturated fat and cholesterol, both of which have been attributed to an increase in cardiovascular disease.

Conventional wisdom states you should not eat too many eggs in one day due to the high cholesterol content. Likewise, over-indulgence in burgers and steaks has been discouraged for the same reason. However, today many health experts are reversing this opinion. We are learning that eggs, red meat and other foods that are high in cholesterol are not the harbingers of death they were once believed to be. Instead, sugar, carbohydrates and trans fats are the true villains.

Cholesterol is essential for the body. It is a major component of cell membranes and is used to make important molecules such as hormones, fat-soluble vitamins and bile acids to help you digest your food. Also, the body naturally creates cholesterol in amounts much larger than what you can eat. So avoiding foods that are high in cholesterol will not affect your blood cholesterol levels very much.

Dental Health

More than half the world's population suffers from some form of gum disease. However, if you are able to catch it early you can stop its progression and, in many cases, reverse its damaging effects.

Proper diet is critical. Even if you visit your dentist every 3-6 months, the care they give is rarely going to extend beyond a few weeks. It is your day to day habits that most impact your dental health. And what food group poses the biggest risk to your teeth? If you guessed carbohydrates then a gold star for you.

Carbs quickly turn into sugar, which creates a range of oral bacteria. This is what causes tooth decay and gum problems. Eliminating refined carbohydrates and sugars is the key to reclaiming your oral health.

A meat-based diet will provide you with coenzymes, collagen, catechins, vitamin C, beta carotene and omega 3s, all of which will protect your teeth and gums. These can be found in foods such as salmon or other fatty fish, grass-fed beef, chicken and bone broth.

Diabetes

If you have diabetes, then you understand the fine line you must walk when it comes to dietary choices.

Sugar in the blood comes from the food we eat and carbohydrates turn into sugar as soon as they reach the stomach. This means sugar (soda, fruit juice, candy) and starch (bread, pasta, rice, potatoes) have to be off the menu.

When you avoid carbs and consume only fatty meats, eggs and cheese, your blood sugar levels will remain low and your hemoglobin A1C level will fall back into a normal range. This is because you are not constantly spiking glucose in the body and forcing your over-worked pancreas to secrete insulin over and over again.

The woeful carbohydrate-rich dietary advice currently given to diabetics is based on the old fear of naturally fatty foods. There are no quality studies showing that a carbohydrate-rich diet is beneficial.

When Swedish experts recently examined the medical evidence, they did not find any scientific studies validating advice for a low-fat and whole grain-rich diet. However, they did find evidence that a LCHF (Low Carb High Fat) diet is better for blood sugar and weight control than today's low-fat advice (Dietary Treatment for Obesity report by the Swedish Council on Health Technology Assessment).

Vision

Several studies have shown that the fish oil found in tuna, salmon, trout, sardines, anchovies, herring and mackerel can help to reverse dry eye and other vision problems (Archives of Ophthalmology).

Beef is high in zinc, which has been connected to better long-term eye health (Mayo Clinic). It has been shown to delay the process of macular degeneration and age-related sight loss. The eyes and the retinas, in particular, contain high levels of zinc so any foods that contain a good dose of it will be of benefit to your eyes.

The Carnivore Diet In Detail

In some respects, the carnivore diet is simplicity itself. You cannot eat anything that did not originate from an animal. This can include typical meat sources such as from cows, fish, pigs and chickens, but you are also welcome to sample more exotic options, which we will look at later in the book.

Here is a list of carnivore-compliant foods and drinks.

Foods allowed on the carnivore diet

- Organ meats
- Poultry
- Fish
- Meat
- Eggs
- Lard
- Bone marrow
- Butter
- Salt and pepper

Beverages allowed on the carnivore diet

- Water
- Coffee (unsweetened and black)
- Tea (unsweetened)
- Bone Broth

Foods some people can tolerate on the carnivore diet

- Milk
- Yogurt
- Cheese

Foods not allowed on the carnivore diet

- Vegetables
- Fruit
- Seeds
- Nuts
- Legumes
- Bread
- Pasta
- Grains

Butter, particularly the grass-fed variety, is fine, while eggs and cheeses are usually acceptable also. However, we would ask you to begin the carnivore diet with just meat, butter to cook with and plain water to drink for 30 days. This will give you all the key benefits of the carnivore diet and is a fantastic elimination diet. Once you have established this baseline of health, vitality and weight loss, you can then add in eggs and cheese and monitor their effects on your body using your daily journal, which we will come to.

For most people, eggs and cheese pose no problems and make a welcome addition to the diet that allows for more varied and interesting meals. However, if your body has a problem processing lactose or egg protein then you might want to forgo one or both of them. The beauty of the carnivore diet is that once you have been on the diet for a while, your body will start to feel healthier, have more energy and in turn will be better able to cope with breaking down the components of food. At this point you can better determine whether or not you would like to add certain food groups or keep to the core basic plan, as you are seeing the results you desire.

On the carnivore diet you will be eating a lot of

fatty meats and parts of animals you might not have tried before, such as the liver or tongue, so you will be getting all the nutrients that your body needs. Do not be overly concerned if certain additional foods are off-limits to you. The key is to find the dietary choices that allow you to become the most vibrant and healthy version of yourself.

All this talk of food restriction may seem extreme and a little overwhelming at first, especially considering the ever-expanding range of foods that we have easy access to in the modern world. But keep in mind that this diet is rising in popularity globally for a reason and, moreover, it has been practiced in parts of the world for hundreds upon hundreds of years. That is because it works in transforming lives for the better.

Many dieters will start the carnivore diet after doing the paleo or ketogenic diet — other diets comparable to this one but which allow for a wider variety of foods. The carnivore diet's high-protein, low-carbohydrate features makes it especially attractive to those looking to lose weight fast without excessive exercise or calorie counting.

Do Not Fear Fat

If one of your primary goals is to lose weight, your initial assumption might be to cut back on foods with high fat content. That just seems logical, and you cannot fault someone for assuming that this is the correct way to proceed based on all the low-fat diet dogma out there. Less fat in the food will equal less fat in and on our bodies, right? Wrong.

Fat in your food is not what makes you fat. In fact, fat in the diet encourages the body to burn its own fat stores through a process known as ketosis, which we look at in more detail. Carbohydrates are the real culprit behind weight gain and all the negative health consequences that come with it. When people eat food containing carbohydrates, the digestive system breaks them down into sugar, which enters the blood stream. As blood sugar levels rise, the pancreas produces insulin, a hormone that prompts cells to absorb blood sugar for energy and storage. The result is an expanding waistline and a whole host of health issues that come along with it.

By way of an example, let us look at the livestock industry. Cattle farmers want to raise their cattle and get them to market as fast as possible. This means they need to put meat on their bones quickly. So what do they feed their cattle? It is certainly not butter, bacon or any other fats or meat. Instead, they feed their livestock a steady diet of grains. Sure enough, the weight of the cows quickly starts to increase. This is because the body of a mammal will naturally take any sugars produced from the grains it digests and store it as fat.

By cutting out carbohydrates, you are cutting out the fuel for fat storage. Your body now has to use its own fat stores to provide energy for your daily activity, which will see weight and excess fat starting to drop off you. This will result in a lean, athletic physique and reduced risk of developing the myriad health complications association with excess weight and stored visceral fat in the body.

Easy Does It

You can start this diet gradually. The shift you will have to undergo is not just nutritional, but mental as well (we have tips for this later in the book). As you start to cut out non-meat foods from your diet, you will also be cutting out calories. On the one hand, this is great for fat loss. However, we do not want to take the calorie deficit too far, or we will end up under-fed with a lack of energy. A good way to replace some of the lost calories is with fattier cuts of meat. Remember, we do not have to fear fat any more.

Have you ever been on a diet and could not stick to it because you were always craving the sugar, the salt and savoriness of the traditional foods you love? Cravings can be your body's way of telling you it needs something, that the food you are currently eating is not sufficient in some way. When you consume fat, you can stave off those cravings a lot easier. Fat helps you to feel fuller and more satisfied for longer, as well as providing you with clean calories that do not cause an insulin spike in the body.

Nutrient Needs

Uninformed dieticians and nutritionists are quick to point out that if you cut carbohydrates from your diet, you will be missing out on the essential nutrition they contain. While it is true that grains and other plant-based foods do contain many macro and micronutrients that our bodies need, they are certainly not the only source of these nutrients.

Our ancestors were not eating an abundance of carbohydrates, so why do we need to now? Processed and high-carb food can be produced inexpensively and in huge quantities by the global food conglomerates, resulting in billions of dollars a year in profits for them. It is no wonder they are marketed so aggressively. Do not become a cog in the giant money-making machine of the food industry. Reclaim your diet and reclaim your health.

To succeed on this diet you will need discipline and time. Many false assumptions about the carnivore lifestyle come from individuals who try it for a few days without giving their body enough time to adjust adequately. They are then disgruntled when they do not immediately see every single one of the touted benefits manifesting.

It is important to keep in mind that everyone has a different body, and people will react differently when it comes to the speed of results and adaption to fat burning. Also, some will find it hard and some will find it easy to maintain this style of eating for long periods of time. Generally, however, you need to try it for at least thirty days before you will consistently see the upsides and can make a fair assessment of whether the diet is working for you.

Think Outside The Box

Going carnivore may require you to change your normal food choices quite radically, and you could find yourself in front of a plate of things that you might never have considered eating before. Aside from the usual meats we are all accustomed to, do not shy away from exotic options such as:

- Buffalo
- Elk
- Goat
- Alligator
- Frog

You can look to other parts of the world for inspiration. For example, in the Middle East, they happily eat camel meat. In Africa, they have a plentiful supply of wild boar, and in Asia, you might find lizards on the menu! Now, you do not necessarily need to eat all, or any, of these things. The point is to keep your mind open as to the definition and options for meat consumption. Keeping your mind open to new ideas will give you more variety in your diet, so you will not become bored. Even if you love steak, you might not want to eat it every day, so learning to try new things and adding variety can help you to stick to the diet for the long term.

Foods To Avoid

We have already discussed the meaning of the word "carnivore" and it certainly means no fruits or vegetables allowed, plain and simple. You will find that most carnivores will agree with this definition, but there are a few things outside of the meat category that carnivores can and do enjoy.

As we have stated before, the ideal way to start the diet is in the strictest form — meat, butter and water for 30 days. This immediately eliminates all potential allergens and a whole host of foods that can potentially disrupt the gut and spike your insulin levels. Meat and water will give you the best results but it is perfectly understandable that for many this is not a sustainable way to eat from a psychological perspective. The best diet is always the one that you can stick to long term.

So some carnivores will permit cheeses, eggs and garnishes. This would be things like using garlic and herbs in cooking, topping meat with cheese and eating eggs for breakfast. Though eggs and cheese come from the animal family, many people have trouble processing them, while others have no issues whatsoever. If you find you can reintroduce them into your diet without affecting the positive results you have obtained from the stricter carnivore diet, then by all means include them.

The carnivore concept is about as easy as it gets, eating only animal foods. So every part of your meal should be derived from living creatures that at one time walked, crawled, swam, or flew around the earth. Other than that, there are no hard and stringent rules to follow. You do not have to worry about counting calories nor do you have to measure portion sizes. When you are hungry, you eat. If you are not, do not.

Your meat selection could include steaks, burgers, hams, poultry of all kinds, fish and wild game for starters. Once you have become accustomed to these foods, you might occasionally want to try some of the more exotic meats such as buffalo or crocodile. The diet is pretty basic in its design.

Now let's examine a few other food groups and see if they are compatible with the carnivore diet.

Oils

If you are not regularly in the kitchen cooking, you might not think too much about the oils contained in your foods. You walk down the aisle in the grocery store and you wonder what all those different oils are actually for. But on the carnivore diet, you can only use oils derived from animals. That means coconut oil, peanut oil, sesame oil or olive oil are all off limits. You can cook your meats in butter and the renderings from other meats. So you can save your bacon fat or the drippings from that baked roast you had earlier. These add a deeper and richer flavor to your meat that can be very satisfying. You can also use grass-fed butter to replace the regular oils that you use.

The oils you want to avoid are probably the most commonly used in other diets. For example, there is a lot of attention in the media being given to olive oil and coconut oil, but on the carnivore diet you want to avoid them completely. Also, definitely steer away from vegetable oils, margarine, soybean, sesame, safflower, rice bran, canola, peanut, palm, hemp and corn oils. There are a lot more that could be added to this list, so as a general rule of thumb, look at the source. If it did not come from an animal, you do not want it on your plate or in your food.

Fruits

Fruits are a very popular food choice for most people, and there is a wide variety of them to choose from. They add a burst of sweetness in the mouth that is far less harmful than the processed deserts we tend to crave. But on the carnivore diet you want to avoid them. The sugar they contain in the form of fructose will have a big impact on your blood glucose levels and hinder your attempts to lose weight.

Vegetables

Quite often when people suffer from digestive issues, it is the result of the grains, legumes, vegetables and nuts they eat. These are a key sources of phytic acid, an anti-nutrient that can interfere with the body's ability to absorb iron and zinc. If you are planning on going strict carnivore, which you should be at the beginning, then completely eliminate vegetables from your diet. However, vegetables can be added to bone broth for a bit more body and flavor (we will cover this later in the book). But never consume vegetables directly.

Dairy

One of the main reasons carnivores avoid dairy is because it often triggers allergies. Dairy, while it is an animal product (derived from an animal), makes many people feel less than their best after consuming it. It is ultimately up to you if you would like to add a little cheese to your meal, but if it gives you digestive problems then it is best to do without it. Here is where your daily journal, which you will learn about soon, is invaluable in tracking its effects on your body, energy levels and overall mood.

Soft Drinks And Alcohol

You definitely want to avoid soft drinks and alcohol on a carnivore diet. These are almost always laden with sugar, which will automatically counteract any benefits you receive from the diet. Sorry guys, that means you will have to give up your beer, wine and afternoon aperitif. These are one of the easiest ways to throw off the results you hope to gain and derail your progress. The next chapter looks at beverages in detail.

Artificial Sweeteners

Not only do sweeteners come from plants and so do not fit into the carnivore diet, they are also synthetically made, which means that they are not something the body can adapt to easily, if at all. You will find them in packages with labels that say "low calories", "light/lite", "diet", "reduced-sugar" or "no sugar added". They may seem like they are a healthy option, but when consumed in even small doses they could contribute to weight gain, trigger cravings for more sweet foods, cause blood sugar levels to be erratic and have a negative impact on your gut bacteria.

Just the mere fact that they are not found in nature should be enough to discourage you from wanting to use them. They are not a natural part of any diet. If you are using artificial sweeteners now, there is a good chance that you will experience some withdrawal symptoms when you stop using them, but those should go away after a week or two. Then you will wonder why you ever felt you needed them.

Sugar And Desserts

Even natural sugars can cause complications with the carnivore diet. If you are struggling with weight and health issues that are affecting your blood glucose levels, it is probably because of the amount of sugars you take in. In the past, sugar was not a regular part of any diet in any society, and on the rare occasions it was consumed, it was never to the extent that people consume it today. It is best to avoid it as much as possible, on any diet.

Once you have been on the carnivore diet for a while, you will find that you do not crave sweetness anymore. In the meantime, you have to suck it up when it comes to sugars. It is a plain and simple NO.

Deli Meats

Interestingly enough, deli meats would logically be considered carnivore compliant, but there is a good reason to avoid them. Deli meats are usually made from a combination of meats ground up and pressed together. Many deli meat manufacturers use plant-based filler ingredients to bind these meats together. As a result, they are not considered 100 per cent meat. For that reason, it is best to avoid all deli meats unless you know exactly what the ingredients are and how they might affect you. Some dedicated carnivores will make their own deli meats and sausages so that they are completely sure of what they are eating.

The carnivore diet does not have to be difficult nor does it have to be painful. There are no hard and fast rules that dictate exactly how you should eat. If you always keep in mind that the primary focus is to eat only animal-based products, all the smaller details should fall into place.

What To Drink

Drinks can be a controversial topic on the carnivore diet. Some dieters feel they can maintain their normal drinking habits without any change whatsoever, while others feel they have to cut out absolutely everything out except for water.

If you frequently visit fast-food restaurants or eat on the go a lot, then you are likely consuming a lot of soft drinks, which are full of sugar, something you definitely want to avoid on the carnivore diet. These drinks will slow down any possible health benefits you hope to gain and can actually start to erode your health. Drinking them will be contrary to anything you hope to achieve on the diet.

Diet soft drinks are also a no-no. It may surprise you to know that these "zero carb" drinks can be as addictive as taking drugs. This is because they are loaded with artificial sweeteners, which we have discussed earlier. Also, artificial sweeteners tend to raise insulin levels in much the same way as real sugar. Your body does not understand that this is a synthetic chemical and not the real deal. So just because it says zero calories or carbs does not mean it is good for you.

Back To Basics

The number one choice beverage on the carnivore diet is, you've guessed it, plain water. It should always be your first choice when you need something to wet the palate. This actually does not just apply to the carnivore diet, but should apply to any dietary plan you create. Many medical problems can be improved significantly if people would just drink more water to stay hydrated and flush out toxins. Water is the only beverage in our history that was consumed by every generation since mankind's beginning. And remember, the carnivore diet is about getting back in touch with our roots.

You should drink water according to your thirst. Experts often recommend that you should drink at least eight glasses a day, but since all people are different, your specific needs for water can also vary. Just like you should consume your meals when your body asks for fuel, you want to take the same view of water. If you are thirsty or feel you are dehydrated, drink water.

However, it is important to understand that sometimes your body is telling you it is dehydrated, but you do not necessarily recognize the signs. Your need for water can appear in a wide range of symptoms that you might not readily identify. You may need to drink more water if any of the following conditions appear:

- You have bad breath. When your body is low on water, one of the first things it stops producing is saliva. If you do not have enough saliva, bacteria will continue to grow in your mouth, causing you to have bad breath.
- Dry skin. If you are really low on water, your skin will lose much of its moisture, sometimes leaving you looking flushed or drained.
- If you are really dehydrated, your need for water can become apparent through muscle cramps. A lack of water can cause your core body temperature to rise, which will automatically cause the muscles to work harder, leading to the cramps.
- Fever and chills: You may have unexplained fever or chills. When the

fever is high for no apparent reason, it is usually because of dehydration. The higher the fever, the more water you need.
- Cravings for sweets: Dehydration can also be the source of your food cravings. When the body's water supply is limited, it can be hard on internal organs like the liver, which relies heavily on water to release glycogen and other body fluids when you need them. The result will be a strange craving for certain foods, especially sweets. While this condition can trigger a wide variety of cravings, the body's call for sweets is a sign that it is struggling to break down the glycogen so it can release more glucose into your bloodstream. It is a common sign of thirst that most people fail to recognize. So the next time you have a craving for a candy bar, reach for a tall glass of water instead.
- You might also get headaches when you need water. Even a very mild case of dehydration can cause headaches and even migraines in some instances. If you have no idea what is causing your headache, first try to drink some water. In many cases, the pain will go away as soon

as your body fluids have been elevated enough for proper function to resume.

So when you are feeling thirsty water should always be your first choice. It is okay to drink a cup of black coffee or tea but try drinking a full glass of water before reaching for these options. You will be glad you did, and your body will thank you for it.

Coffee and Tea

This may not be a surprise to you, but the one drink that people have the hardest time doing without is coffee. It is a popular mainstay in nearly every country in the world, especially in the mornings. The good news is that because it carries zero calories, it is an acceptable beverage for almost everyone who is on the carnivore diet. However, you would want to exercise caution if you are predisposed to any type of sensitivity to caffeine, which many people have. Remember that your body will be going through an adjustment phase at the beginning of the diet and how it responds to that morning cup of Joe may not be the same. Pay close attention, and if you sense any type of negative reaction such as extra sensitivity to caffiene and jiteriness, stop drinking it or reduce your intake.

The same can be said for tea. Because there are hundreds of different types of teas in the world, it may be difficult to predict how the particular tea you drink will affect you on your new diet. Many teas have proven healing qualities, but they also contain caffeine. Again, be aware of any impact that it is having on you that is out of the ordinary. Here is where your daily journal will prove invaluable.

Broth Benefits

Bone broth is a favorite choice for carnivore dieters. It is essentially the bones of animals and certain spices boiled in water to create a soup. It is very easy for carnivores to make due to the fact they consume so much meat and therefore have many bones leftover.

It can be made from just about any bones - fish or mammal - and is both tasty and a nutritional powerhouse. Bone broth is rich in minerals that support the immune system and contains healing compounds such as collagen, glutamine, glycine and proline. The collagen in bone broth also heals your gut lining and soothes any intestinal inflammation.

If you do not have any bones to hand you can go to your local butcher and ask for a few soup bones. They are also sometimes available in packs at the supermarket.

To make the broth, place the bones in a pot and cover with water. Allow it to cook over a low heat until the bones become soft or the marrow starts to come out. The nutrients will be in the marrow so try to get as much of it out as you can from the bone. You can add a few vegetables to the pot for a little flavor, but make sure that you strain those out before you drink the broth.

For a plain broth, you might cook the mix for a few hours, while for a stronger broth the pot can be left to simmer for the entire day. Some even cook the mix for two or three days — but that might be a little extreme for our purposes. The longer the time on the stove, the more minerals and nutrients that are extracted from the bones, so you get a much richer flavor and more nourishment from the same starting ingredients.

Regardless of which option you choose, your body will get an abundance of nutrients from the marrow, including proteins, collagen and gelatin. These are then broken down into smaller amino acids that contribute to gut health, resilience to illness and endurance. It really is good health in a cup.

Putting It All Together

Make no mistake, you will have to make changes when it comes to consuming beverages. It may not come as a surprise that you will have to cut out any Coke-a-day habit and forget about the Big Gulp from your local 7-11 store. However, there are many other drinks you will also want to avoid. We focus our beverage intake on these staples:

- Water
- Coffee (unsweetened and black)
- Tea (unsweetened)
- Bone Broth

Bottom line? If you want to get a clear idea of how life would be going full-on carnivore, you will drink only water and bone broth. However, if you want to keep your coffee or tea, that is acceptable as long as you monitor the effects. Whatever you decide, make sure you avoid consuming any type of artificial sweeteners as these will definitely counteract the positive results you hope to achieve.

How To Start The Diet

Making the switch to the carnivore diet does not have to be difficult. Yes, you will have to give up some of your favorite go-to foods that you have enjoyed for years, but you will have more of other things that up until now you have been told were bad for you. So maybe you say no to potato chips and cookies, but you can say yes to more steaks, hamburgers (minus the bun) and bacon.

In truth, your success on the carnivore diet will depend a great deal on how motivated you are. If you are already meat lover, making the transition may be an adjustment for the first few days but, after the first week or so, you should have slipped right into the new dietary routine.

One tip that has been very effective in helping people to switch over is to surround yourself with those who are sharing the same journey. It helps a lot if your family is willing to join you on this new venture. If not, there are meat lover communities everywhere. Join an online carnivore group the first chance you get (a recommended resource list is provided at the back of this book). You will find scores of supporters, recipes and tips that will help you to overcome any obstacles that you might be facing.

For most people, the degree of difficulty in adapting to the diet will depend on where you start from. If you are starting from a typical high-carb diet, you will have a bit more of a struggle. It would wrong and misleading to suggest otherwise.

You will probably start to experience something that is often referred to in the low-carb and no-carb world as "keto flu". This is range of common flu-like symptoms that occur when you cut your carbohydrates. Basically, you might think of these effects as carb withdrawal symptoms. In essence, your body starts to complain when it is no longer getting the sugar high it has become accustomed to. The good news is that it is only temporary and usually goes away over a period of just a few weeks. But you need to hang on in there and ride it out.

On the other hand, if you are transitioning to the carnivore diet from a cleaner diet such as the paleo, ketogenic or Atkins diet, your chances of getting the keto flu will be much lower and your transition will go a lot more smoothly.

Symptoms Of Keto Flu

It is referred to as the flu because the symptoms you will be feeling will be very similar to what you might experience when you really do have the flu. Only this is not the result of any type of viral infection. So do not be surprised if you start off feeling fatigued, experience light headaches or body aches. Less common symptoms include feeling irritable, low energy and difficulty concentrating.

If you find that you are dealing with a case of keto flu, here are a few tips that can help you manage it. They are also great tips in general for starting on the carnivore diet.

Make A Gradual Transition

While you may be excited about making the switch, it is important that you ease into the diet. By starting off slowly, you can lower the extent of your symptoms. Going all meat can be a drastic change, not just nutritionally but psychologically as well. So there is no need to drop all your foods cold-turkey. You can start by making one meal in the day carnivore, and then once you become accustomed to that you can move on to the next one. One of the easiest meals to start with is breakfast. Some bacon or baked salmon would be a quick and easy choice.

Another way to ease into the diet is to replace each component of a meal one at a time. For example, if your breakfast consists of eggs, bacon, toast, cereal and juice, you can start by replacing the toast with a bigger serving of eggs. The following day, you would replace your cereal — maybe with an extra slice of bacon. Then the next day substitute the fruit.

There is nothing wrong with cutting everything non-meat out cold turkey, but just like quitting smoking, it is not something that everyone can do easily. So do not feel too discouraged if you find that the going is tough. The key is to see it through.

Start At The Right Time

You do not want to start the diet when you have a lot of distractions that could get in your way. A good option is to choose a time when you can spend a few days at home. This could be on the weekend, during a work break, or while you are on vacation. These are the times when you are most relaxed and have fewer obligations to get in the way. If you start during these more relaxed times, you can more easily slip into your new eating routine without distractions. Also, if you come down with a case of keto flu, it will be much easier to handle when you are not under work or study stress.

Stock Up

You want to make it easy on yourself to make the transition. That means first getting rid of all those tempting non-compliant foods that you are drawn to and stocking up on a good variety of meats. The more options you have on hand and quick access to, the less likely it is that you will reach for something off-limits when you are hungry.

Carve Out More Time For Rest

It is true that you will get a nice burst of energy when you go carnivore, but you may find that in the beginning you will need to squeeze in a little more rest. This does not mean that you have to add a few extra hours to your sleep during the night, but squeezing in some nap time in the middle of the day certainly will not hurt.

Your body is going to be making a major transition — burning fat for fuel rather than glucose — and it will need time to adjust. Your muscles, mind and nerves will be trying to figure out what is going on initially, and that may put a toll on your system. So allowing for more time to relax could help you to ease into this new program. Once your brain and body figure out that everything is fine and that they will be supplied with good clean nutrition, it will be smoother sailing.

Come In With A Balanced Frame Of Mind

Keep in mind that you are making a pretty extreme change. It is likely that you have a very specific goal in mind, but be realistic about your expectations. If you are looking to lose weight, have an open mind about how much you will lose. Going into the diet expecting to drop ten to fifteen pounds in a week will quickly lead to discouragement and loss of enthusiasm if your rate of progress is slower. As we have said before, the diet will give different results in different people and you will not know what kind of outcome you will experience until you actually start it.

Get Family And Friends On Board

There is safety in numbers, and the more people who know about your goal and what you expect to achieve, the more support and social accountability you will have. Let your friends know that you are starting something new and ask them to help you stay on the straight and narrow. You will inevitably come across naysayers who will think your diet is plain crazy, but sometimes all it takes to get them on board is to ask them to help monitor your progress. People like to feel useful and involved. So rather than engaging the skeptics in a lengthy debate that will end up with both of you feeling frustrated and angry, just humbly ask them for help in your endeavor. They will soon learn firsthand that you will not die from eating just meat.

What's In A Name?

If you feel that you cannot get those around you on board, you may be able to introduce the diet in another way. Rather than telling them you are going full-on caveman carnivore, consider describing it in a different way. "I'm going on a no-carb diet", or "I'm attempting an elimination diet". These types of phrases sound much more reasonable than "I'm going to be a prehistoric meat eater". They may still feel a little uneasy, but the gentler terms sound far less threatening than "all-meat diet" or "carnivore".

Plan Ahead

There is no denying that eating meat can be quite costly, especially if you do not budget properly. When you walk into a supermarket and find a single cut of steak costing upwards of ten dollars, it can be an unnerving experience. But if you plan ahead, you can bring down the expense. Compare prices of local supermarkets to see where the best deals are to be had. Also, do not exclude local butchers, which could offer surprisingly good value for money. Also consider buying a large freezer and then ordering your meat in bulk. Yes, there is an upfront cost, but a larger freezer will allow you to buy and store a whole side of beef or pork. The cost per pound of meat then works out significantly cheaper than buying individual pieces of meat.

Learn To Cook

If you are not a regular home cook, you will quickly find that there are very few eateries out there that will offer you compliant all-meat menus. Plus, you cannot vouch for the quality of meat you are presented with in restaurants. The more you are able to prepare your own meals, the more satisfied you will be with what you are eating and the more cost-effective the diet will be. Learning how to perfectly grill a steak or grind up your own meat for meatballs or hamburger patties can be immensely satisfying and motivating

Hydrate

As mentioned previously, staying hydrated is one of the most important parts of the carnivore diet. Even with good nutrition, people often fail to keep themselves adequately hydrated. Water is the life force of your cells and it is even more important to stay hydrated when your body is going through a major change.

Not only is water important for maintaining healthy cells in the body, it will also help to curb any carb cravings you might have when you first start the diet. Whenever you get a hankering for something that you should not have, drink a tall glass of water, and soon that craving will disappear. It really works. When you are fully hydrated, your body will be satisfied and satiated for longer, and your desire for forbidden food and drinks will soon disappear.

Don't Shy Away From Fat

Though we have discussed this before, it is important to reiterate the point. For years we have been told to eat only lean cuts of meat because eating fat is bad for your health. However, new research is now showing that consuming fat does not cause you to gain fat. In fact, it is quite the opposite. When you consume a nice fatty piece of meat, you not only get more nutritional value, but the fat content will encourage ketosis, which in turn will burn your own fat stores.

So you do not have to throw away the skin of the chicken. Bacon, in all its fatty glory, can grace your plate every morning, and you are more than welcome to enjoy the rich and deep flavors of a fully marbleized steak. The added good news is that eating this way will save you money, as fatty pieces of meat are usually the least expensive.

But there are other forms of fat you can indulge in, too. For example, you can now swap out your processed margarine with creamy grass-fed butter, ghee, lard and cheese. Remember, we advise you to stick to meat and water initially and track your results. But you can add these foods back into your diet if they are not affecting your weight loss or health goals and your digestion remains good. You will add more flavor to your meals rather than having the same things day after day. In fact, the more fat you include in your diet, the easier it will be for you to stick to it as nothing is as satiating to the body as fat.

When you cook your meats, make sure you use a pan that will collect all the drippings so you can use them later. There is nothing like fried eggs in the morning, but that flavor gets even richer when they are fried in the drippings from the bacon. There is no longer any reason to fear fat. The added flavors will have you looking forward to every meal with anticipation.

Don't Be Afraid Of Salt

Seasoning your meat will be the key to adding to its variety and desirability. Do not be afraid to use salt in your dishes, especially sea salt, which is a far healthier option than standard table salt. It not only makes the meat taste good, but it also helps to keep your body's electrolytes in balance. This will be an essential ingredient to every meal. Without it, you could find yourself enduring cramping in the muscles that might cause you to think twice about your new endeavor. As a general rule of thumb, you want to make sure that your body is always well hydrated and that your food is salted to prevent this from happening. Good fats, salts and proper hydration are also the keys to preventing sugar and carbohydrate cravings.

When you first start a low-carb or no-carb diet, your body will flush out much of the excess fluids you have been retaining. This is a good thing for weight loss and achieving a lean and athletic look. However, as these fluids are flushed out, they will also take with them important electrolytes. By adding a little extra salt to your diet, you can slow down this process, preventing those muscle cramps or any other potentially negative side-effects.

Muscle cramping can also be the result of a lack of magnesium or potassium. By adding a little extra salt to your meal (especially the kind that contains both sodium and chloride), you can prevent it from happening. Getting the right amount of potassium can be a little trickier since to receive the daily recommended allowance you would need to consume about three pounds of meat a day. For that, you might want to consider taking a potassium supplement until your body adjusts to its new nutrition plan.

Keep A Journal

You will want to keep a record of your progress and the corresponding foods you are consuming. If fact, this is essential. Keeping a journal can help to keep you motivated as you see the results you desire on paper. What do you want out of the carnivore diet? These are the metrics you need to track. This could include weight loss, more muscle definition, more energy, a lessening of arthritic symptoms or simply a greater feeling of well-being.

The act of writing down everything you eat and seeing the corresponding results will inspire you keep with the diet or make changes if things are not quite on track. You will be able to see at a glance what works and what does not, and you can make the necessary adjustments immediately rather than waiting until the end of the week or month to figure out what is working. The scale not budging? You might need to decrease your daily calories. Feeling lethargic? You might need to increase the amount of water you drink and up your salt intake.

You can supplement your written record with pictures. Take a "before picture" prior to embarking on the diet and then periodically take pictures of your physique as you chart your progress. As a matter of fact, it is a good idea to stop reading this book right now and take your before picture! Even if you are not ready to start the diet today, it will serve as a reminder of your starting point and why you want to bring change into your life. It may even motivate you to get started sooner.

Join Groups

As mentioned before, in today's connected society you have a world of potential supporters and friends out there who are doing the same thing as you. They have the same trepidations, questions, doubts and are facing the same daily challenges. Take advantage of this community. Whether you are on Facebook, YouTube, Twitter or Instagram, there is a carnivore society waiting for you to join the party — see the resources section at the back of this book for specific recommendations. If you spend enough time interacting with those who have already jumped the hurdles you are currently facing, you will have the wisdom you need to point you in the right direction.

Build Flexibility Into Your Routine

When your diet consists of eating only meat, there is no doubt that initially it can get boring quickly. It helps in the beginning to have one day in the week to go off and eat whatever you want. This will take much of the stress out of such a limited diet, but will not do you any serious damage. If you find you miss the taste of your favorite veggies, choose to have them on a flex day. Or maybe you just cannot resist getting a slice of cheesecake when you are out with your friends. Save that privilege for an occasional flex day to keep life a little more bearable at the outset.

Make sure that you schedule your flex day rather than just move it around randomly. For example, if you have decided to have your flex day on a Saturday but when Saturday rolls around you are not inclined to go off the diet, do not assume that now you can have it on Sunday or Tuesday. Instead, understand that if you do not go flex on Saturday, you will have to wait until the following Saturday to indulge. This will keep you from losing your rhythm so you will stick to the program for longer. Remember, eventually we want to phase out flex days altogether so you are 100 per cent carnivore and reaping the full benefits of the diet.

Make no mistake, going from a standard modern

diet to eating exclusively meat will represent a challenge, but if you can implement these different strategies you will find that making the transition will be a lot easier. The hardest part of the carnivore diet is getting started. So the more of these tips you implement at the beginning, the faster you will adjust to your new nutrition plan. Once you are through the adjustment period, it should be much smoother going.

Making A Meal Plan

When you start the diet it helps to have a meal plan in place, so you do not have to over-think what you are going to do each time you are hungry. The meal plan you start with may not be one you stick to long-term, but the key is to get started and then you can make the necessary adjustments so that your meals will better fit your lifestyle and tastes.

When you create your meal plan, make sure that you incorporate a good deal of variety in it, especially during the first ten days. You may start off liking steak, but if you are eating it every day, you may soon tire of it and will fall off the wagon.

The purpose of having a meal plan is to help ease your transition without the added stress of not knowing what to cook or eat. Below are a few suggestions to get you started. We begin with food options for one day on the strict carnivore diet where it is just meat. This is followed by a 4-day guide to more flexible carnivore eating, where you can add more variety.

STRICT DIET

Breakfast
5 bacon slices
(You may also choose to skip breakfast and fast until lunch if you are incorporating intermittent fasting, which we will come to soon).

Lunch
Rib-eye steak, or chicken livers, seasoned with salt and pepper.

Snack
1 cup bone broth

Dinner
Three hamburger patties seasoned with cayenne, onion powder, garlic powder, salt and pepper, or two large salmon fillets.

LOOSER DIET

Day 1:

Breakfast
3 eggs cooked in organic butter from grass-fed cows
4 slices of bacon

2 slices of cheese
1 cup of black coffee or tea

Lunch
½ lb. ground beef prepared with ½ cup of cheese

Dinner
12 oz. steak prepared with organic butter

Day 2:

Breakfast
Ham and Omelet

Lunch
1 chicken breast cooked with a ½ cup of parmesan cheese
2 slices of bacon
1 cup of bone broth

Dinner
Classic Roast Chicken

Day 3:

Breakfast
Pork Sausage and Eggs

Lunch
12 oz. steak prepared with organic butter

Dinner
Two fish fillets (tilapia, catfish, red snapper)
1 cup of bone broth
2 slices of cheese

Day 4:

Breakfast
Same as Day 1

Lunch
½ lb. ground turkey cooked with ½ cup of parmesan cheese

Dinner
Simple Baked Salmon

As you can see, the meals are pretty basic and simple to cook, but since you are going to be cooking most of them yourself, it is still important that you have them planned out well ahead of time.

Finally, a few additional tips to help you.

- Plan for snacks between meals. You may not need them, but carry around a bit of cheese or jerky just in case you get a craving for something before the next meal.
- Remember your goal is zero carbs, so anytime you have a craving for carbs (usually happens at the beginning of the diet), substitute the carbs for fat.
- Avoid lean meats and opt for fattier cuts for more satiation.

Keep in mind that once you get started, your body is going to find its own rhythm. As it does, you may find that you are not inclined to eat all three meals in the day. Do not force feed yourself. If you are not hungry, do not eat. It is as simple as that. Work in harmony with your body, not against it.

Supercharge Your Results

So far we have gone into detail on what you should eat on the carnivore diet, but have you ever considered when you should eat? There is an approach to meal timing called "intermittent fasting" that could boost your results on the carnivore diet.

It is actually a technique that can be paired with any diet, even a standard American one, as it promotes better insulin control and is a painless way to eat fewer calories. So incorporating intermittent fasting (IF) into your day can boost the health optimizing aspects of the carnivore diet and is especially useful if your primary goal is to achieve weight loss quickly.

The core idea behind IF is that you will go without food for a large part of the day. There will only be a few hours in which you will be allowed to eat. This time frame is called your "eating window".

In nature, it is not realistic or even attainable to eat every three or four hours as we humans do. The body can very easily go for twelve hours or more without consuming calories. This is especially true on the carnivore diet, because animal-based foods are extremely nutrient dense and satiating, making fasting that much easier.

But you might be wondering just why you should limit the number of hours in which you are eating each day. After all, you have already cut out all of the bad foods from your diet. You no longer consume sugar, grains, processed food, low-quality carbohydrates or all the other things that could potentially cause you harm.

With IF, you eat the same amount of food you would normally eat, but you will only consume it during the set hours you have chosen. Most people have an eating window of eight hours while others will restrict it down to just four. There are even some who will choose to only eat every other day — but that is a bit extreme for our purposes!

At first glance, this process might seem strange and even ridiculous if you are still consuming the same amount of food (and thus calories) as you would normally. However, when you look at the science behind IF you will understand there is a method to this seeming madness. If your goal is to lose weight, this is a great way to put your fat loss on the fast track. When you fast, your body processes all of the food you have eaten so far in the day. When those food sources are completely digested, your body will drain its supply of glucose reserves (the fuel it uses for energy), forcing the body to switch over to burning its own fat for fuel. This process, as we learnt before, is called ketosis.

However, the body will never burn its own fat if there is plenty of food calories available. It will only switch to burning fat if all other sources of fuel have been depleted. If you are eating every few hours throughout the day, you are continually adding to your supply of stored energy, so your body will never have a reason to even consider using your stored fat for fuel.

Think of it this way. Assume you have a house that you need to keep warm in the winter time. Your heating system runs on electricity so when the temperature drops, you automatically switch on the electric heater and soon your home is nice and toasty. But, one day, a storm passes through and, for a time, you experience a power outage. How will you keep your house warm? If you have a fireplace or a wood-burning stove, you would simply toss some firewood in there, add a little kindling and strike a match. Soon your house is nice and toasty again.

In the body, glucose (electricity) is the primary method of energy, but fasting creates that power outage. When there is no more glucose, the body still needs to run so it switches over to burning fat instead (wood). By not feeding your body for extended periods of time, it forces the body to find alternative forms of energy. When glucose is gone, what is left is your own fat. Intermittent fasting actually helps you to tap into your natural fat stores much faster.

In addition to weight loss, intermittent fasting has many other benefits that you may not be aware of. Consider these points:

- It lowers your risk of disease: Because it encourages fat loss, your risk of diseases resulting from obesity is minimized. Also, because it slows down the aging process and helps to keep a healthy flow of blood to the brain (through a process known as autophagy), your risk of neurodegenerative diseases is also minimized, protecting you from

conditions like Alzheimer's and Parkinson's.
- Through IF, you protect the nerve cells of the brain, causing slower degeneration than you would otherwise experience. It causes your body to go through a process of clearing away old damaged cells so that new ones can be generated.
- It helps to improve memory and facilitates faster learning.
- It eases depression and several other mood disorders.
- It lowers cholesterol, slows down the progress of cancers (which love glucose) and keeps the body's cells resilient.

So whether you are looking to accelerate your weight loss, or you are interested in some of the other health benefits listed, IF is scientifically proven to work.

When it comes to intermittent fasting, do not be afraid to experiment to find the right eating window for you. Some people are not able to fast every day of the week, while others can fast every day without a second thought. Do not get too caught up worrying about the rules. The key is to go as long as possible without eating so your body can shift into ketosis.

Just remember to do the following:

- Fast for at least twelve hours a day.
- Only drink water during the fast (no food of any kind).
- Only eat if you are hungry after the fasting period.
- Listen to your body: if you find that your blood sugar is dropping fast or you get any other signs that things are not going well, stop the fast.

By adding intermittent fasting to your regimen, you can accelerate the benefits you will already be receiving from the carnivore diet. You will find that you have more energy and your overall health markers will improve.

Are There Any Downsides?

While many critics claim that the carnivore diet is merely a passing fad, the evidence is clear that societies throughout history have used it with success. This is probably one of the main reasons why it has such strong appeal among so many today. Humans have been eating meat for millions of years. It is rich in calories and nutrient dense. Even if our society today is not completely meat oriented, there are few on this planet that go completely without it.

To put it simply, meat is our baseline food, and everything else that goes on our plate is a complement to the main feature. It is programmed into our DNA. Organizations and so-called health gurus work hard to try to convince us to stay away from it, but there is a deeply embedded pull of our ancestors that will not allow us to let it go completely.

While there are many false arguments that too much meat is bad for your heart, bowels and general health, the truth is that good healthy meat is nutritious and beneficial. You never hear about people being allergic to meat, but they are to grains, gluten and dairy. All that being said, this book would be a disservice to you if we did not raise some of the concerns over a carnivore style of eating. Here are some points to bear in mind.

Cholesterol

One of the biggest concerns when it comes to an all-meat diet is the potential to raise cholesterol levels. There is no question that meat contains a great deal of cholesterol and saturated fat. Its consumption can encourage the liver to produce more cholesterol than the body typically needs in order to function.

For example, a small 3-ounce portion of prime rib has around 14 grams of fat, 6 of which is purely saturated fat, and about 75 milligrams of cholesterol. This is more than the daily recommended allowance as outlined by the American Heart Association.

Yes, the carnivore diet works in lowering body fat, lowering blood pressure, helping you to sleep better, and even improving digestion, but there is no doubt that it can increase cholesterol. But is this a dangerous outcome? If you are feeling good and all of your other health markers are on point, will a higher cholesterol level really lead to a heart attack?

When you have high cholesterol, the knee-jerk reaction is usually to treat the condition with drugs. The American Heart Association regularly issues warnings about elevated cholesterol, but in recent years many of the studies they have based these warnings on have been called into question. Let's look at the facts.

Cholesterol is an essential component needed for every cell in the body. In fact, 25 percent of our cholesterol is used by the brain and the central nervous system to keep us functioning at peak performance. Our bodies produce copious amounts of it, just in case we run out. This means that our cholesterol levels are constantly changing. Add to that, every year people with low cholesterol are suffering heart attacks. Heart disease requires a number of factors, not just one.

In 2017, academics and cardiologists from 17 countries reviewed 19 previous heart disease studies, involving 68,000 patients. They found no link between heart disease and high LDL cholesterol — in fact there were hints that those with higher cholesterol levels actually survived for longer. Their findings were published in the prestigious BMJ Open journal.

One of the authors, cardiologist Dr Aseem Malhotra, said: "The scientific evidence clearly reveals that we must stop fear-mongering when it comes to cholesterol and heart disease and focus instead on insulin resistance, the most important risk factor as a precursor to many chronic diseases."

And what causes insulin resistance? Sugar, grains and carbs. Not meat.

Nitrates

Nitrites are frequently added to processed meats like bacon, ham, sausages and hot dogs. They function as preservatives, helping to prevent the growth of harmful bacteria. However, there is some evidence that nitrites can damage cells and also morph into molecules that cause cancer. The best way to avoid this problem is to keep foods such as smoked bacon, sausages, cold cuts, salami, jerky and hams to a minimum. A good alternative is meats that are fresh on the bone, as they pose much less of a risk to your health.

Mercury

Fish can be an important part of a healthy diet. It contains high-quality protein and other essential nutrients, as well good omega-3 fatty acids. However, almost all fish (and shellfish) contains traces of mercury. Generally, the risk of mercury poisoning by eating fish is not a major health concern. Yet, some fish and shellfish contain higher levels of mercury that may cause harm when eaten in very large quantities.

It is best to avoid shark, swordfish, king mackerel or tilefish. Instead opt for shrimp, canned light tuna, salmon, pollock and catfish, as they have been shown to contain the least amount of mercury.

Risk Factors

Before you start on the carnivore diet, it is important that you look closely at your health. If you have existing medical conditions, you should consult with your doctor before embarking on this or any other nutrition plan. This will help you to know which dietary approaches are suitable for you, what potential risks you face personally, and whether or not this diet could be of benefit to you.

Who Should Avoid The Diet?

Like any diet that encourages ketosis, the carnivore diet can put a stress on the body during the adaption phase. You may wish to spread the carnivore message to your children and loved ones, but you should hold off on initiating those who are still growing and developing, or women who are carrying children in pregnancy.

A carnivore diet is not recommended in children under eighteen as they would find it very difficult to adhere to, particularly if they take meals at school. Also, as their young bodies and brains are growing at a rapid pace they can process glucose much better than full-grown adults and it will not generally result in obesity. You can still advise them to avoid processed and junk foods and introduce them to some of the recipes found in the carnivore diet to ensure high levels of good protein.

As mentioned in the previous chapter, asking your doctor for a physical assessment and general blood work before beginning the diet is a good idea to ensure you do not have any unknown underlying health conditions like diabetes or kidney problems. Both of these conditions would restrict the safe diet options that are available to you.

Those who have liver, pancreas or kidney issues should not attempt the carnivore diet, as it could put too much stress on the body and potentially worsen your pre-existing problems. Muscular dystrophy is sometimes known to cause complications, albeit only rarely, and those who have a history of eating disorders may also struggle with this diet as it could act as a trigger to restart their condition.

The above stipulations are not meant to scare you. The carnivore diet is generally very safe and advantageous to your health, assuming you have no pre-existing conditions that could be exacerbated by a high-protein all-meat diet. Healthy adults who are looking to lose weight and feel good will find great success going carnivore, so long as they continue to monitor their health closely and listen to their body and its needs.

Walk On The Wild Side

It is true to say that those who opt to go carnivore often live life on the more adventurous side. To the skeptics, it is a shocking diet and you will need some degree of independent thought and even bravery to embrace it. You must not be afraid to step out of the norm and try something different.

In this same spirit, let's look at some exotic meats that you may not ordinarily find on your plate. However, on the carnivore diet they can add some much-welcome variety and novelty. Most of us have tasted a little wild meat or game from time to time, maybe at a restaurant. But few of us do this on a regular basis. We tend to always go back to the regular staples such as beef, pork, chicken, fish, and the occasional duck or goose. But there are some good reasons why you would want to sample more wild meats.

For a start, wild meats have become far more accessible of late. Today, you can walk into a US gourmet restaurant and order a plate of ostrich, go down to Mexico and order up a large dish of goat birria, or take a bite out of an alligator in the

Florida wetlands. While you may scrunch your nose up at some of these ideas, you might be surprised to learn that not only are these meats quite tasty, but they can be very good for you, too.

Most of these wild animals are not bred in captivity or in a controlled environment, so they tend to be higher in protein and are not subject to the same antibiotics and other chemicals that farm animals could be exposed to. Plus, consuming these wilder meats can actually be good for the environment. Growing livestock populations on farms cuts down on our water resources, consumes more and more land, and contributes to global warming.

So do not be afraid to take a walk on the wild side and try something new. Below are some exotic meat options you might want to sample. They are all available at specialty butcher shops across the United States and much of the rest of the world. In some cases, you might have to ask your butcher to have the meat ordered in for you. Remember, buying in bulk will cut down the cost in the long run.

Bison (3 oz. serving)
145 calories
5g fat
2g saturated fat
24g protein
73mg cholesterol

Yes, the mighty bison still lives and breathes in the vast plains of the United States. Interestingly enough, according to the USDA's National Nutrient Database, it is a much healthier option than standard beef with fewer calories and a whopping four times more omega-3 fats. Whenever possible, make your burgers with bison rather than beef. You will also get a much bigger burst of flavor. You can prepare bison in pretty much the same way as you would any beef recipe, but expect the taste to be a tad sweeter with a deeper and richer tone.

Rabbit (3 oz. serving)
167 calories
7g fat
2g saturated fat
25g protein
70mg cholesterol

If you are looking for a sweet, tender piece of meat, rabbit is a delicious option. You can find rabbit in many supermarkets across the country, but often you have to go to a butcher if you want to buy it. It is commonly served in countries like New Zealand, Belgium and China. It has a very mild flavor and its nutritional profile is second to none in the meat world. One serving contains more protein than any type of beef or chicken you can find. It is loaded with iron and essential minerals such as phosphorous and potassium. Get a few whole rabbits and keep them in your freezer for an efficient way to consume this meat.

Ostrich (3.5 oz. serving)
132 Calories
3g fat
1g saturated fat
24g protein
79mg cholesterol

Another delicate meat that will surprise your taste-buds is ostrich. While it is a bird, it does not taste like any bird you have eaten before. Its meat is more red than white and is very similar in texture and flavor to a steak rather than a chicken drumstick. Ostrich meat has considerably more B vitamins than other types of meat, which your body needs to maintain a healthy metabolism and brain.

Venison (4 oz. serving)
162 calories
3g fat
2g saturated fat
31g protein
96mg cholesterol

Do you like hunting? This is an easy choice for anyone who does not mind bagging their own game. Venison (deer meat) has a taste and texture similar to beef, but with just a little more punch to it. It is extremely lean, so its calorie content is considerably lower than that of beef. It has less fat and cholesterol, too. One serving of venison will give you more iron and protein than you would get from your normal steak or hamburger. If you are not inclined to go hunting, most butchers have large quantities of the meat on hand.

Elk (3.5 oz. serving)
124 calories
1.5g fat
0.5 g saturated fat
26g protein
62mg cholesterol

Elk is quite a large animal, much larger than a deer in fact, but its flavor is quite mild and a little sweeter. Its nutritional profile is quite similar to deer, but it has more vitamin B-12 (essential for nerve and blood cells) than you can expect from deer meat. In fact, one small serving gives you 100 percent of your total daily requirements in addition to high doses of iron, thiamine, phosphorous, zinc and riboflavin.

Quail (4 oz. serving)
193 calories
12g fat
3g saturated fat
21g protein
73mg cholesterol

If you are not familiar with the name quail, you might know this bird as the partridge or the bobwhite, depending on where you are in the world. Quail is often served roasted in the same way as chicken or turkey, but it is much smaller. A single quail is probably only enough for one person, but it provides plenty of protein, iron, zinc and magnesium in every bite. This small bird has a much stronger flavor than chicken or turkey, but if you prepare it with your standard spices and flavorings, it can be difficult to tell the difference.

Goat (3 oz. serving)
122 calories
2.5g fat
1g saturated fat
23g protein
64mg cholesterol

Lamb's older cousin is a nutritional powerhouse well worth taking a bite out of. Not only does it have fewer calories per serving, but it also has less fat than beef or chicken. It is a sustainable meat source as the animals do not need to be fed grains of any kind, so you can easily keep one in your yard and let it feed on your grass. It has a nice savory taste but bold at the same time. It is great to use in stews and recipes that require long simmering times.

Alligator (3.5 oz. serving)
232 calories
4g fat
0g saturated fat
46g protein

Alligator is not only low in calories but high in protein. You can serve it in a wide variety of ways but if you choose to deep-fry it, you are going to lose much of its nutritional benefits. This white meat has a light grainy texture that can be compared to pork or chicken. While you can eat almost every part of the alligator, the most flavorful and tender part is the tail, which has been compared to veal.

Incorporating exotic meats and wild game is a good way to keep your diet interesting, so you can stick with it longer and reap the many benefits of being a carnivore.

Advice On Eating Out

Eating an all-meat diet is pretty straight forward when you are at home and in command of your own kitchen. You know everything that goes into every dish and you can prepare exactly what you want without worry. However, challenges present themselves when you have to go out to eat. It is not reasonable to expect that you will never want to join your family and friends for an occasional dinner out on the town. This diet should not turn you into a hermit.

When dining out, you first need to approach the situation with the right mindset. Just looking at all the options on the menu can get your mouth watering as you recall all the foods that you once indulged in. Temptation can easily get the better of you and, before you know it, you have a plate full of high-carb goodies in front of you, but you know in your heart of hearts that this is the wrong way to go.

Being tempted is only human. After all, these were the foods that you indulged in for many years. Now, as you find yourself in a social situation where everyone else is indulging, it is tempting to throw caution to the wind "just this once".

The good news is that it is very possible to go out and not fall into such traps, but you need a plan of action. Simply follow a few basic rules and mentally prepare before you go out, so you know exactly what you are going to do. Here are the key steps.

Make A Plan

If you know what restaurant you are going to, go online and look at their menu. It is easier to prepare if you know what you are in for. Make your carnivore-compliant menu decisions ahead of time — before the waiter has a chance to tempt you on the actual day with his detailed descriptions of what you will be missing out on.

Set The Scene

If you know you have a weakness for pasta, then try to steer your group away from Italian restaurants. In fact, it can be very helpful if you ask to choose the restaurant rather than allowing it to be a group decision, especially if the majority of the group are not on a low-carb eating plan. Types of restaurants that tend to be very carb heavy are Italian, Chinese and Mexican. These have much fewer low-carb/carnivore options to choose from. However, if you find yourself in one of these places, there are ways around this problem. Keep reading.

Don't Be Afraid To Ask For What You Want

Remember, you are the customer. Order with confidence and let the waiter know that you are on a special diet. Make it clear what you want and what you do not want. Think of it in the same way as having a medical condition. Imagine a person coming in with a peanut allergy and being told that they will have to have a dish with peanut sauce, no matter what!

Do not ever be afraid to ask for a steak, pork ribs or piece of chicken completely on its own without any sides, sauces or garnishes. With the surge in popularity of low-carb diets, restaurants are now used to such request and can easily cater for your needs. But you have to speak up.

How To Order

While restaurant menus can vary in many ways, most will usually have special diet sections or an a la carte menu to order from.

Look for meats that are not breaded or coated with anything. Ideally, you want meats that are grilled, broiled or roasted. These are less likely to have things added in the cooking process that you do not want to eat. If the dish comes with a salad, rice or bread, just tell the staff to leave it off the plate - do not allow yourself to be tempted. Better yet, you might be able to trade some of those side dishes with others in your party for an extra piece of succulent meat!

Order burgers without the bun. You could also ask for eggs in lieu of the normal sides that come with a meal. Make it a habit to look for substitutes wherever possible.

As long as you have a plan and the willpower to see it through, it is more than possible to spend enjoyable times with your friends and family while still complying with your diet. Let's say it again, plan, plan and plan again!

Frequently Asked Questions

Chances are, when you first heard about the carnivore diet, you had a lot of questions and doubts. You probably heard how fruits and vegetables are essential to give you the nutrients you need to maintain good health. You probably thought about all the warnings about fat in meat and how it can destroy your arteries and health.

If you were thinking along those lines, you were not alone. There is no question that eating carnivore-style can be considered an extreme diet, and it is not for everyone. If you are still undecided, then the following questions and answers might be able to put your mind at ease.

Medical science is slowly but surely coming around to the correct view that fat and protein are not responsible for our modern health woes. The blame lies at the door of sugar and cheap carbohydrates.

It is up to you to decide whether or not this is the right step for you. If after reading this book you are still in doubt, then talk with your medical practitioner to see if there are any other causes for concern that you need to be aware of. Then take all the knowledge you have accumulated and weigh it up before making a final decision. You need to make an informed choice that feels right for you.

Q: Should I eat the carnivore diet all year round?

A: Yes, for sure. Keep in mind that the Inuit and the Maasai, who traditionally practice this diet year-round, do not succumb to modern western diseases. Some people keep an all-meat diet plan on the backburner for when their medical conditions flare up and they need an anti-inflammatory eating protocol to tackle their symptoms. But if the diet shows benefits, why not enjoy those benefits throughout the year instead of just occasionally?

Q. Will I get all my vitamins and nutrients if I go pure carnivore?

As research evolves, it is becoming clear that the recommended daily allowances for various nutrients are not a static number. How much nutrition you need depends on a variety of factors including your age, weight, gender, activity level and diet. So, for some people, the carnivore diet will give them all the nutrition they need, while for others there may be a need to take additional supplements to satisfy their requirements. This would have been the case whatever dietary approach they followed.

It is important to note that researchers have recently discovered that those on a carb-heavy diet tend to require more additional nutrients than those who are not. In general, however, if you are eating good quality fresh meats you should be able to get everything necessary, particularly if you are taking in an adequate number of calories. In addition, the vitamins and minerals you get from animal products are much more easily absorbed into the body than those that are received from synthetic sources.

It is recommended that you have blood work done a few weeks into your diet to ensure that everything is where it should be.

Q. How much should I eat?

The carnivore diet does not require you to count,

measure or calculate in order to get a finely balanced meal. The general rule of thumb is to eat when you are hungry and then stop when you are full. You should follow your body's cues and let it dictate to you how much you need to eat.

That being said, most beginner carnivore dieters fail to eat enough. Because meat normally does not make up the majority of our meals, it can be difficult to adjust to eating so much of it. We are just not used to larger portion sizes. If you find your energy levels slipping, that is your signal to increase food intake.

As stated earlier, if you find that you are struggling eating all-meat right away, consider easing into the diet. Have a regular meal with all the sides but start by eating your meat first.

How much you eat will also depend on how much energy you need throughout the day. If you are young and active, you will need to eat more to keep up your stamina, but if you are living a more sedentary life, then you will need less. Let your body guide you.

Q. What about fiber?

We have been told for years that fiber is essential to keep our digestive system functioning properly. However, fiber is not always your best friend. In many cases, it can interact with blood sugar, especially when consuming too many carbs, to cause stomach upsets. Interestingly enough, you need more fiber when you are eating carbs, so if you have eliminated them from your diet then extra fiber is not necessary.

Fiber creates bulk, which can sometimes make it difficult for your body to eliminate waste. Those on the carnivore diet have reported no problems with digestion or elimination.

Q. Should I only eat grass-fed meat?

Ideally, grass-fed meat would be your first choice. These are animals that are not fed any grains so the meat will be more natural without any risk of hormones or other additives being passed on to you. It usually has higher concentrations of some nutrients: antioxidants, some vitamins, a kind of fat called conjugated linoleic acid and the long-chain omega-3 fats mostly found in fish. That said, grass-fed meat can be quite costly and may not be an option for many people. In such cases, eating more fish or eggs (if you tolerate them well) would be a good option.

Also, the assumption that all animals that are not grass-fed have been abused is not true. There are many ranchers who take very good care of their animals; they are not crowded into filthy warehouses where there is not much room to breathe or move. So do not assume that because the animal has not been fed-grass, or is not free-range, that it has suffered or been mistreated. Buy the meats you can find and afford, but make sure they are fresh and from a reputable supplier.

Conclusion

Well done for making it to the end of *The Carnivore Diet Bible*. I sincerely hope it was informative, enlightening and has provided you with the tools to change your diet — and life — for the better.

Odds are that when you first heard about the carnivore diet you were very skeptical. There is no question that it challenges many of the established beliefs we have been taught from childhood about health and nutrition.

However, thousands of people around the world have seen the dramatic effects of eliminating cheap processed carbs and sugars, and returning to the natural food source we were meant to consume. They have seen inflammation leave their bodies, allergies subside and excess weight drop off, allowing them to reclaim their health and once again live a full life.

For decades we have followed the dietary advice of government health bodies when it comes to our nutritional choices. But what has the "balanced plate" including fruits, vegetables and so-called "healthy carbohydrates" brought us? A global epidemic of obesity, rampant autoimmune diseases, no let up in heart disease deaths and increasing diabetes rates. Does it not make sense to try a radical approach to change our health outcomes?

The bottom line is that we, as individuals, are responsible for our health and what we put into our bodies. We cannot hand this responsibility over to anyone else — our lives literally depend on it.

So it is time to step up to the plate, embrace you ancestral roots and make the diet changes to set your life on a healthier path. If you choose embark on the carnivore diet, then welcome aboard. You are in very good company.

Wishing the very best of health to you and your family.

Stephen Baker

30 Easy Carnivore Recipes

By now you will no doubt have in-depth knowledge of exactly what the carnivore diet involves and why it can be so great for your health. However, it can still be difficult to begin or maintain due to the restrictions when it comes to food choices. It is such a world away from standard western diets.

If you are going carnivore after being on a paleo or ketogenic diet previously, this challenge might not be so hard, as you are already used to eating all that high-protein, high-fat goodness. However, if you are starting out on the journey you might need some guidance and inspiration.

In the following pages you will find 30 delicious recipes that cover breakfast, lunch, dinner and even snack options.

We encourage you to start the carnivore diet with just meat and water to reap the full health benefits and kick start your journey to health and fat loss. The following recipes are for when you are looking to expand your carnivore-compliant food options. As always, it is important to track your food intake via your journal and notice what effect, if any, the dishes are having on your progress.

These recipes may include cheese, eggs and various garnishes and seasonings. However, vegetables are never consumer directly. Feel free to adjust ingredients to suit your tastes and preferences.

Bon appétit!

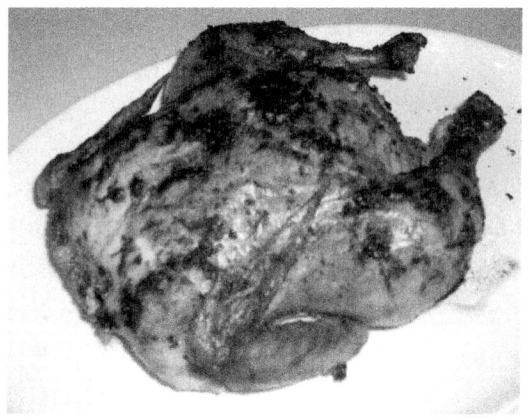

Classic Roast Chicken

Total Prep and Cooking Time: 120 Minutes
Yields: 8 Servings
Nutrition Facts:
Calories: 267
Protein: 28 g
Net Carbs: 0 g
Fat: 16 g

Ingredients

1. One whole chicken
2. Two rosemary sprigs
3. Two cloves of garlic (Seasoning only)
4. One tbsp. salt
5. One tsp. assorted herbs
6. Glass cooking pan

Instructions

1. Let your chicken "rest" from the fridge until it reaches room temperature. It should be lukewarm to the touch.
2. Preheat your oven to 350°F and let it heat during the prep process.
3. Remove any coverings on your chicken and rinse it under cold water to ensure it is clean.
4. Put your chicken on your cooking pan breast-up and fill the cavity with the rosemary sprigs and the cloves of garlic. You do not have to peel them in preparation.
5. Mix the assorted herbs and salt together in a small container.
6. Rub half the seasoning onto the chicken itself.
7. Flip the chicken side-down and repeat and save any leftover seasoning for other meats.
8. Bake for ninety minutes or until skin is browned. Meat should be white and not pink to indicate if it's done or not.
9. Serve immediately and drizzle the cooking fat from the pan on top.

A whole chicken roast is a meal that humans have consumed for thousands of years. In this recipe, the stuffing will provide a great flavor to the meat while the drizzled cooking fat will add an extra kick to elevate this meal. Chicken is also a perfect dish to make once and spread out across your week in the form of cold cuts.

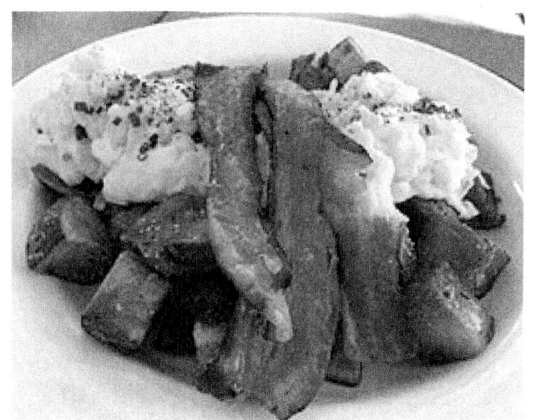

Eggs and Bacon

Total Prep and Cooking Time: 15 Minutes
Yields: 4 Servings
Nutrition Facts:
Calories: 272
Protein: 15 g
Net Carbs: 1 g
Fat: 22 g

Ingredients

1. Eight eggs
2. Five ounces of organic bacon slices
3. Frying pan with lid

Instructions

1. Fry all your bacon in one pan and rotate out if you need more room. The fat in the pan from your cooking will help the bacon to cook, and you should not remove it.
2. Crack your eggs into the bacon grease once you have removed all the bacon, and cook them however you like.
    a. For over easy: After a few minutes of frying, flip the eggs over and cook again for another few minutes.
    b. For sunny side up: Cover the pan with the lid and do not flip them over.
3. Remove the eggs once cooked, serve with bacon and enjoy.

Bacon and eggs is a dish as old as time, and the perfect breakfast to start the day. The bacon fat is going to add flavor to your eggs. If you would rather be a stricter carnivore, you can forgo the eggs and instead fry more bacon to satisfy your appetite.

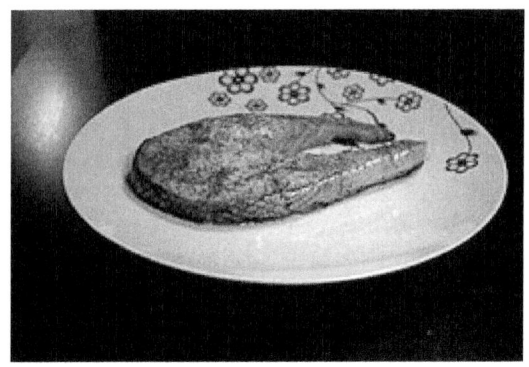

Simple Salmon

Total Prep and Cooking Time: 15 Minutes
Yields: 4 Servings
Nutrition Facts:
Calories: 304
Protein: 36.6 g
Net Carbs: 3 g
Fat: 15.7 g

Ingredients

1. Four salmon fillets (six ounces in total)
2. One tbsp. garlic powder
3. One-half tsp. salt
4. Two tbsp. butter
5. One tbsp. dried basil
6. One skillet

Instructions

1. Mix the garlic powder, basil and salt together in a small bowl or container and rub onto the salmon. Save excess for other recipes.
2. Fry in the skillet over medium heat with the butter, around 3–5 minutes each side until the exterior is brown and the insides are fully cooked. Serve with water for a simple dinner.

Salmon is a prime example of simple and healthy eating on the carnivore diet. It is one of the most tender and best-tasting seafood options and is packed with antioxidants and omega-3 goodness. It is also very quick and easy to prepare.

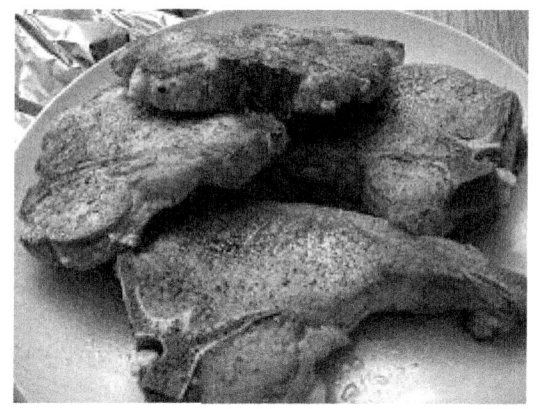

Oven-Baked Pork Ribs

Total Prep and Cooking Time: 190 Minutes
Yields: 3 Servings
Nutrition Facts:
Calories: 440
Protein: 25 g
Net Carbs: 2 g
Fat: 36 g

Ingredients

1. One rack of baby-back ribs (one pound)
2. One tsp. garlic powder
3. One tsp. chili powder
4. One tsp. onion powder
5. Half-tsp. cayenne pepper
6. One tsp. smoked paprika
7. One tsp. salt

8. Parchment paper
9. Baking tray

Instructions

1. Prepare your baking tray with the parchment paper while setting your oven to preheat at 275°F.
2. Mix your seasoning up in a bowl and put aside.
3. Remove the membrane from your ribs on the back side and dry them off.
4. Rub the seasoning mix into the ribs until both sides are completely covered.
5. Put the ribs on your rack and let them cook in your preheated oven for 3 hours.

Pork ribs are a delicious choice for dinner and provide left-overs that keep on giving. This is a good recipe to throw in the oven while you exercise or get some work done, due to the long cook time. You can marinate the ribs overnight in their spices before cooking to get an even deeper flavor.

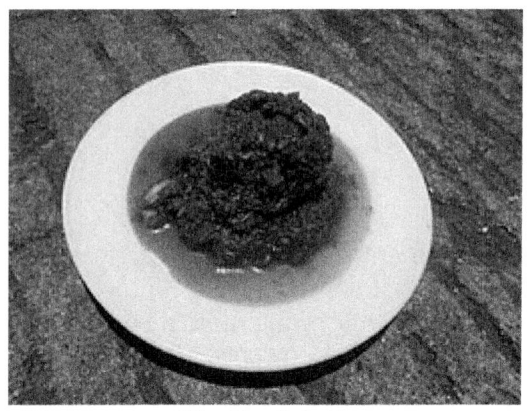

Pulled Chicken

Total Prep and Cooking Time: 6-7 Hours
Yields: 4 Servings
Nutrition Facts:
Calories: 510
Protein: 51.5 g
Net Carbs: 2 g
Fat: 30 g

Ingredients

1. Six boneless and skinless chicken thighs
2. One-third cup of salted butter
3. One-quarter cup red wine vinegar
4. One-quarter cup natural chicken stock
5. Two tbsp. yellow mustard
6. Two tbsp. spiced mustard
7. One tbsp. cumin

8. One tbsp. chili powder
9. Two tbsp. water
10. One tsp. cayenne pepper
11. One stick of butter
12. Crockpot/slow cooker
13. One measuring cup

Instructions

1. Combine your chicken stock, red wine vinegar, mustard, water, chili powder, cumin and cayenne pepper into a measuring cup.
2. Throw either fresh or frozen chicken thighs into the crockpot/slow cooker.
3. Pour your seasoning mix on top.
    a. If you will be going out, add one-third of a cup of butter and set the crockpot to low heat for seven hours. This is to ensure nothing burns, but you still get a fresh meal by the time you are home.
    b. If you will be staying home, let it cook on medium heat for two hours, and proceed with the recipe.
4. Measure out one-third of butter from the stick and let it sit as the chicken cooks, naturally melting.
5. Once two hours have passed, stir the chicken in the pot slightly so all the juices combine and add the room temperature butter. Turn the cooker to

high and cook for three or four more hours.
6. By this point, your chicken should be fully cooked. Shred it with two forks and remove the lid, cooking on high for another forty-five minutes.
7. Stir the chicken and sauce together with a large spoon and serve with fresh coarse sea salt.

If you work a 9-to-5, this is a great dinner option for busy days. By using a slow cooker or a crock pot, you can throw all your carnivore-friendly ingredients in and let it cook while you are away. This recipe really brings out the flavor in the chicken.

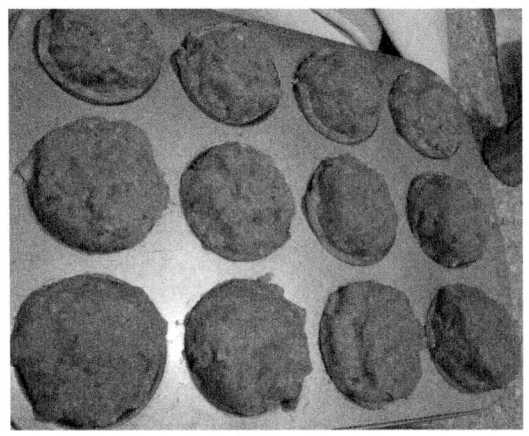

Meat Cupcakes

Total Prep and Cooking Time: 40 Minutes
Yields: 12 Servings
Nutrition Facts:
Calories: 221
Protein: 15 g
Net Carbs: 1 g
Fat: 17.2 g

Ingredients

1. Seven hundred grams of ground beef - low-fat preferably (read why below)
2. Two eggs, lightly beaten
3. Salt and pepper to taste
4. One hundred grams of shredded cheese
5. Two bacon slices (uncooked), diced
6. Muffin/cupcake tins

Instructions

1. Preheat oven to 350°F and let your meat rest after you have taken it out of the fridge until it is room temperature.
2. Combine the beef, eggs, salt, pepper and bacon bits in a bowl, as if you were making meatballs.
3. Place small handfuls of the meat mixture into the tins, just as you would for cupcakes. *If you use beef for this recipe that is too high-fat, it will make a mess in your oven with the grease overflow.*
4. You have the option to cover your meat cupcakes with grated cheese.
5. Cook for thirty minutes and serve as a side or on their own.

These little snacks are perfect for lunches or to be packed away to eat on the go. The compact size means they can be carried around easily.

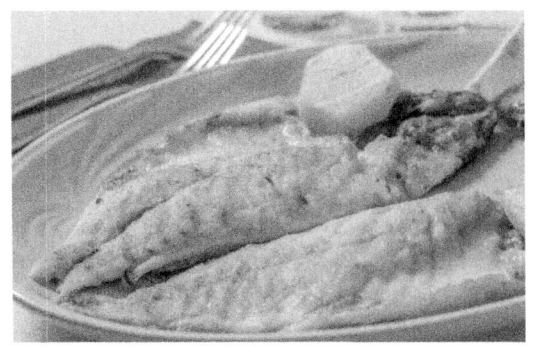

Traditional Cod

Total Prep and Cooking Time: 20 Minutes
Yields: 2 Servings
Nutrition Facts:
Calories: 215
Protein: 37g
Net Carbs: 3 g
Fat: 5 g

Ingredients

1. Ten ounces of wild cod (Preferably freshly caught; four fillets)
2. One egg
3. One tsp. salt
4. One tsp. garlic powder
5. Half-tsp. pepper
6. Cooking sheet

Instructions

1. Preheat your oven to 300°F.
2. Whisk your eggs in a large bowl and soak your fillets of cod in them, one minute each side.
3. Place the cod on the cooking sheet and season.
4. Bake in the oven for 10 minutes. If the fish meat splinters easily with something like a fork, it is done.

This recipe takes less than half an hour to prepare, making it perfect for quick dinners or lunches. Cod is one of the most adaptable fish in terms of flavor and will take on the taste of whatever it is seasoned with. The egg will provide a nice glaze to the fish.

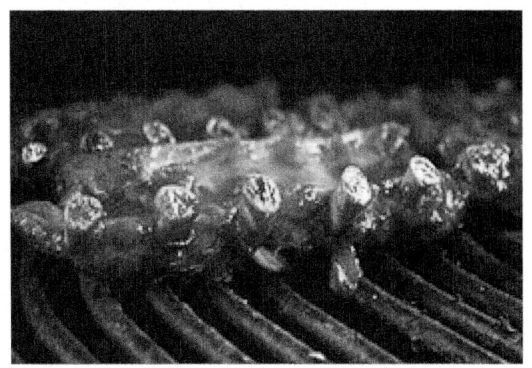

Grill-Smoked Ribs

Total Prep and Cooking Time: 180 Minutes
Yields: 10 Servings
Nutrition Facts:
Calories: 438
Protein: 44 g
Net Carbs: 2 g
Fat: 27 g

Ingredients

1. Five-pound rack of ribs
2. One tbsp. salt
3. One tbsp. paprika
4. One tbsp. garlic powder
5. One tbsp. onion powder
6. One tbsp. chili powder
7. Half-tsp. cayenne pepper

8. Half-tsp. black pepper
9. Smoker box or barbeque.
10. Tinfoil

Instructions

1. Mix up your seasoning in a bowl.
2. Rub the ribs with the mixed seasoning and place it in the tinfoil.
3. Put your tinfoil with the ribs into the grill and let it cook lid-down at 225°F for at least two hours, bone-side down.
4. Serve alone.

A great summer evening dish to serve with friends outdoors. These smoked ribs just fall off the bone and are the perfect dish to enjoy late at night with the meaty smoke in the air.

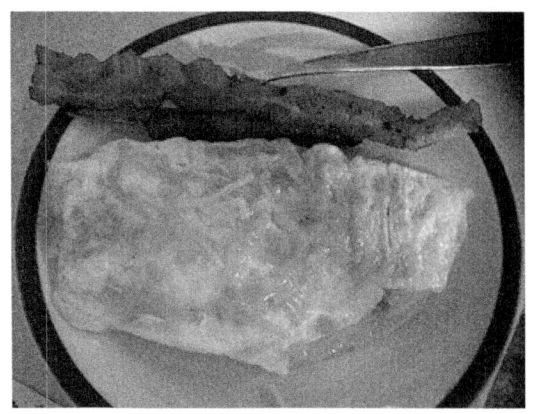

Omelet and Bacon

Total Prep and Cooking Time: 30 Minutes
Yields: 2 Servings
Nutrition Facts:
Calories: 737
Protein: 21 g
Net Carbs: 2 g
Fat: 72 g

Ingredients

1. Four eggs
2. Five ounces of bacon (diced into cubes)
3. Three ounces of butter
4. One tbsp. fresh-chopped cloves
5. Baking dish/frying pan.

Instructions

1. Preheat the oven to 300°F and grease your small frying pan with the butter.
2. Fry the bacon up until crisp and remove from the stove.
3. Whisk your eggs up and add the bacon to the egg mixture.
4. Add salt and pepper to taste.
5. Pour the mix into the oven-safe baking dish and cook for 20 minutes until golden and set.
6. Cool and serve with more bacon if desired. You can also add grated cheese the instant it is out of the oven to let it melt over for extra flavor.

Omelets are a delicious use of eggs on the carnivore diet. This recipe will start your day off with a high-protein boost.

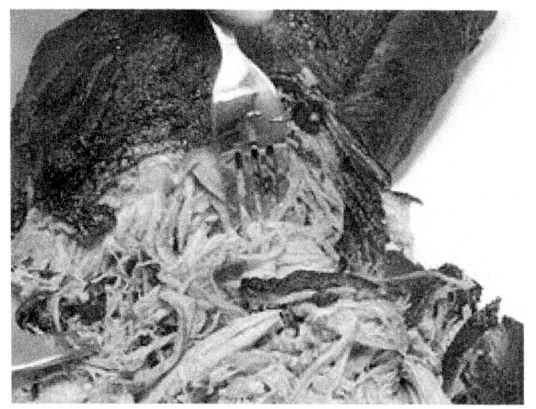

Pulled Beef

Total Prep and Cooking Time: 4 hrs and 5 mins
Yields: 3 Servings
Nutrition Facts:
Calories: 241
Protein: 27 g
Net Carbs: 3 g
Fat: 22 g

Ingredients

1. 2 lbs. of boneless roast beef chuck or round roast
2. 1 cup beef broth
3. 2 tbsp. Worcestershire sauce
4. 1 tbsp. mixed seasoning

Instructions

1. Place roast beef into a slow cooker and add beef broth.
2. Pour Worcestershire sauce over the top of roast and sprinkle with mixed seasoning.
3. Cook roast in slow cooker for 4 hours on high setting (or 6-8 hours on low).
4. Remove from slow cooker with tongs into a serving dish. Break apart lightly with two forks and then add back the gravy in the slow cooker.

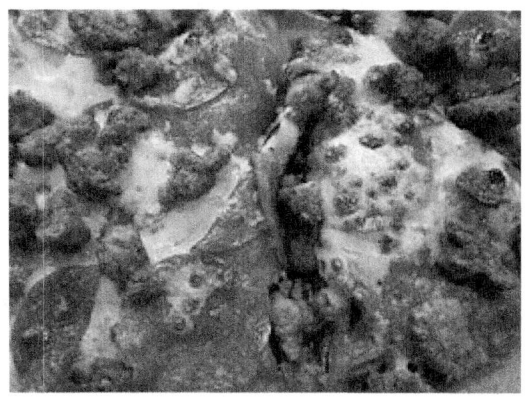

Meat Pizza

Total Prep and Cooking Time: 60 Minutes
Yields: 4 servings
Nutrition Facts:
Calories: 241
Protein: 37 g
Net Carbs: 3 g
Fat: 22 g

Ingredients

1. 1 lb. shredded chicken breast or rotisserie chicken (about 4 cups)
2. 1 cup of shredded mozzarella cheese
3. 2 large eggs
4. Salt and pepper to taste

Instructions

1. Shred the chicken or cut into small ½ inch chunks.
2. Place in a food processor and set to grind.
3. Salt and pepper to taste.
4. Pre-heat the over to 400°F.
5. Line a pizza pan or a baking sheet pan with parchment paper.
6. Thoroughly mix all the ingredients together until well blended.
7. Press the ground chicken down on the parchment paper spreading it out as thin as you can (make sure there are no holes in the dough).
8. Bake for 20 minutes or until you see the edges begin to brown.
9. Top with your favorite pizza toppings (see below) and put back in the oven.
10. Bake for another 10 minutes.

Possible Toppings

Pepperoni

Bacon

Ground beef

Ham

Sausage

Cheese

Shrimp

Chorizo

Chicken
Anchovies
Smoked oysters
Prawns
Tuna

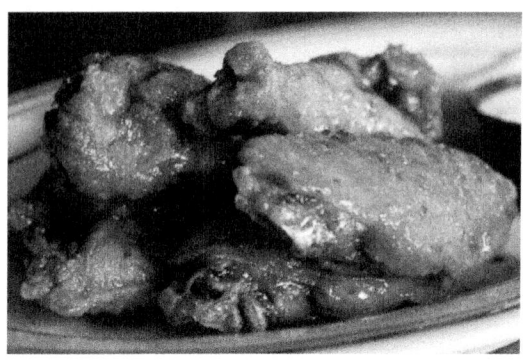

Grilled Chicken Wings

Total Prep and Cooking Time: 30 Minutes
Yields: 12 Servings
Nutrition Facts:
Calories: 181
Protein: 17 g
Net Carbs: 10.1
Fat: 14.6 g

Ingredients

1. 3 lbs. chicken wings, cut at the joints

Sauce Ingredients

1. ¼ cup butter
2. 1 tsp. soy sauce (low carb)
3. ¼ cup hot pepper sauce

Instructions

1. Mix the soy sauce, some water and chicken wings together.
2. Place in a large zip-lock bag and seal.
3. Refrigerate for a minimum of 4 hours or overnight.
4. Preheat your grill to medium heat.
5. Melt the butter in a small saucepan.
6. Stir in the hot pepper sauce.
7. Turn off heat and let rest.
8. Remove the chicken wings from the zip-lock bag and pat dry.
9. Place the wings on a preheated grill, turning occasionally.
10. Cook on medium heat until chicken is well browned.
11. Place grilled wings in a large serving bowl.
12. Pour the butter sauce over them and toss well.

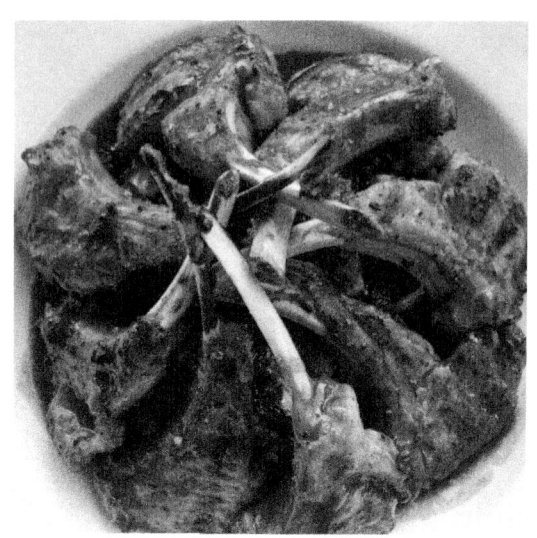

Lamb Chops

Total Prep and Cooking Time: 40 Minutes
Yields: 4 Servings
Nutrition Facts:
Calories: 255
Protein: 14.6 g
Net Carbs: 5 g
Fat: 19.3 g

Ingredients

1. ¾ tsp. dried rosemary
2. ¼ tsp. dried basil
3. ½ tsp. dried thyme

4. Salt and pepper to taste
5. 4 lamb chops ¾ inch thick
6. 1 tbsp. bacon renderings
7. ¾ cup chicken broth
8. 1 tbsp. butter

Instructions

1. In a small mixing bowl, mix the rosemary, basil and thyme.
2. Add the salt and pepper.
3. Rub the mixture onto both sides of the lamb chops.
4. Place them on a plate, cover and let rest for 15 minutes.
5. In a large skillet, heat the bacon renderings over a medium to high heat.
6. Place the lamb chops in the skillet and cook for 3½ minutes on each side or until you have reached your desired level.
7. Remove from heat and keep warm until ready to serve.
8. Stir the chicken broth in the skillet, making sure to scrape any bits of lamb from the bottom of the skillet.
9. Cook over medium-high heat until it has reduced by half (approximately 5 minutes).
10. Remove from heat.
11. Stir in the butter.

12. Pour sauce over the lamb chops and serve.

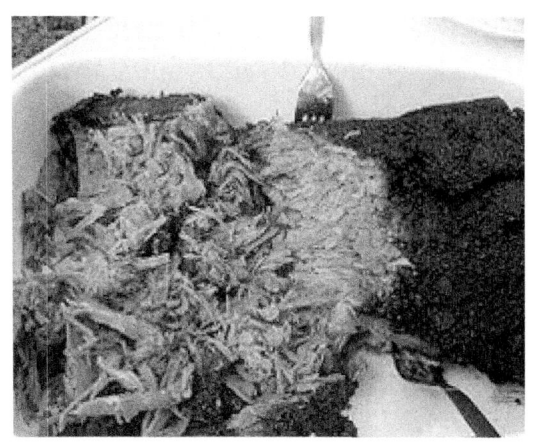

Pulled Pork

Total Prep and Cooking Time: 8 hours 10 Minutes
Yields: 6 Servings
Nutrition Facts:
Calories: 241
Protein: 28 g
Net Carbs: 3 g
Fat: 22 g

Ingredients

1. 4 lbs. pork shoulder roast
2. ½ cup chicken broth
3. ½ cup apple cider vinegar
4. 1 tbsp. Worcestershire sauce
5. 1 ½ tsp. dried thyme

6. 2 minced cloves of garlic
7. 1 tbsp. prepared yellow mustard
8. Butter as needed

Instructions

1. Place the pork roast in a slow cooker and cover with the broth.
2. Stir in all the remaining ingredients except the butter.
3. Cover and cook on high heat until the pork is tender enough to be shredded with a fork (approximately 6 hours).
4. Shred the meat and return to the cooker for 2 hours.
5. Stir the meat in the juices until it is well coated.
6. Serve hot with butter.

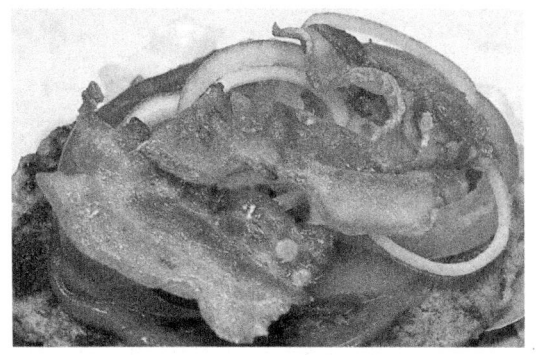

Bacon Burgers

Total Prep and Cooking Time: 40Minutes
Yields: 4 Servings
Nutrition Facts:
Calories: 241
Protein: 33 g
Net Carbs: 3 g
Fat: 23 g

Ingredients

1. 1 lb. ground beef
2. 1 lb. ground buffalo or bison
3. 1 lb. ground lamb
4. 1 lb. ground pork
5. 4 large eggs
6. 1 lb. of bacon

Instructions

1. Heat up the grill to 450°F
2. Pre-heat the oven to 325°F
3. Add all the meat (except bacon) and eggs in a large mixing bowl.
4. Use your hands to make sure it is all mixed thoroughly.
5. Divide the mixture into 4 equal parts and form into tight balls.
6. Flatten each ball into a burger shape approximately 1¼" thick.
7. Salt and pepper to taste.
8. Weave the bacon by placing half of the strips vertically across a baking sheet.
9. Make sure that each strip is touching the one next to it.
10. Lay another strip across each one horizontally.
11. Continue this weaving pattern until you have a single layer of bacon.
12. Take the weaved bacon and place in the oven for 15 minutes.
13. Remove from oven and drain the grease.
14. Return and cook for another 10 minutes.
15. Put the prepared meat patties on the grill and cook for 5-7 minutes on each side.
16. Keep in mind that the thicker the patty, the longer it will take to cook through.
17. Place bacon on top of patties and serve.

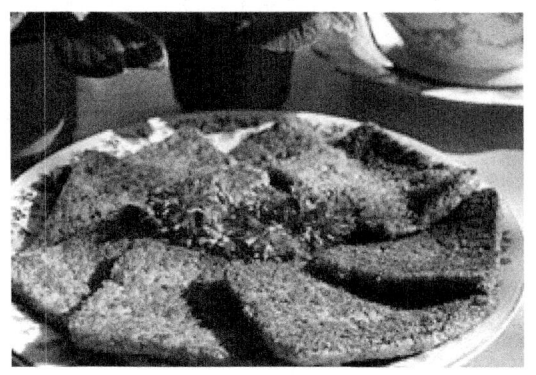

Fried Liver

Total Prep and Cooking Time: 17 Minutes
Yields: 5 Servings
Nutrition Facts:
Calories: 333
Protein: 24.2 g
Net Carbs: 5 g
Fat: 24.4 g

Ingredients

1. 1 lb. beef liver, thinly sliced
2. ½ cup lard
3. 1 clove of crushed garlic
4. 1 tbsp. fresh mint
5. 1 tsp. salt
6. ¼ tsp. fresh ground black pepper

Instructions

1. Pre-heat a large frying pan over medium-high heat.
2. Rinse the liver under cold running water to remove all traces of blood.
3. Pat dry with paper towels.
4. Remove all veins with a sharp knife.
5. Cut crosswise into thin slices.
6. Combine melted lard with garlic, mint, salt and pepper until well-mixed.
7. Brush the liver slices with the mixture.
8. Fry the liver for 5-7 minutes on each side.
9. Remove from heat and serve immediately.

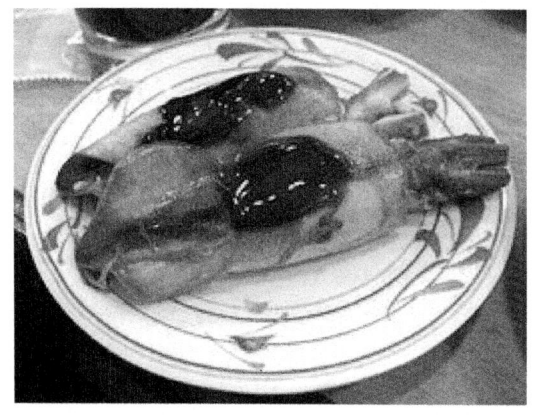

Fresh Oysters

Total Prep and Cooking Time: 15 Minutes
Yields: 2 Servings
Nutrition Facts:
Calories: 600
Protein: 27 g
Net Carbs: 9.2 g
Fat: 33 g

Ingredients

1. 6 oysters

Instructions

1. Rinse the oysters thoroughly in cold water.
2. Do not use a regular kitchen knife to open them as you can easily break off the tip causing injury.
3. With one hand, hold the oyster with the curved side down on a cutting board (keep a folded dish towel between your hand and the oyster shell).
4. Look for the hinge between the top and the bottom shell.
5. Stick the tip of a sturdy knife into the crack (you will have to push hard to get it inside).
6. Pry the top shell off.
7. Season the oyster as desired and eat.

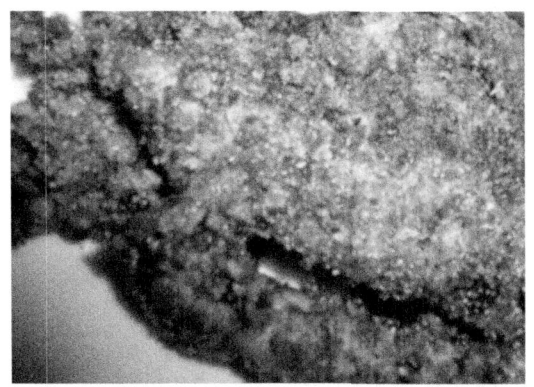

Bacon-Crusted Chicken

Total Prep and Cooking Time: 40 Minutes
Yields: 4 Servings
Nutrition Facts:
Calories: 606
Protein: 45 g
Net Carbs: 3.5 g
Fat: 23 g

Ingredients

1. 4 large chicken breasts
2. ¼ cup mayonnaise
3. 1 ½ cup bacon bits (pre-cooked)
4. 2 cloves minced garlic
5. ¼ tsp. sea salt

Instructions

1. Pre-heat oven to 450°F.
2. Line a baking sheet with foil and grease lightly.
3. In a food processor, pulse the cooked bacon bits with the garlic and sea salt.
4. Transfer the pulsed mixture to a large mixing bowl.
5. In a medium-sized bowl, add the mayonnaise.
6. Coat each chicken breast in the mayonnaise.
7. Roll each coated breast in the bacon bits.
8. Bake for 15-18 minutes or until the chicken is thoroughly cooked and bacon is nice and crispy.

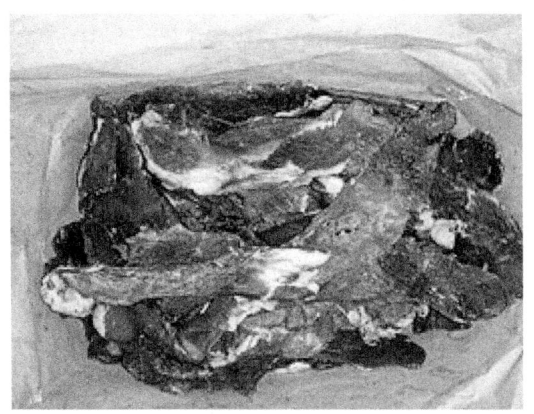

Homemade Jerky

Total Prep and Cooking Time: 6 hours 15 Minutes
Yields: 6 Servings
Nutrition Facts:
Calories: 286
Protein: 32.7 g
Net Carbs: 13.9 g
Fat: 10.5 g

Ingredients

1. ¾ cup Worcestershire sauce
2. ¾ cup soy sauce
3. 1 tbsp. smoked paprika
4. 2 tsp. black pepper
5. 1 tsp. red pepper flakes
6. 1 tsp. garlic powder

7. 2 lbs. thinly sliced beef top round

Instructions

1. Whisk together the Worcestershire sauce, soy sauce, paprika, black pepper, red pepper flakes, garlic powder and onion powder in a large mixing bowl.
2. Add beef to the bowl and make sure it is completely coated with the mixture.
3. Cover the bowl with plastic wrap and place in refrigerator.
4. Let sit for a minimum of 3 hours or overnight if possible.
5. Transfer marinated beef to paper towels and let dry.
6. Arrange the slices on a baking sheet.
7. Bake in the oven until texture is dry and leathery.
8. Cut into bite-sized pieces with scissors.

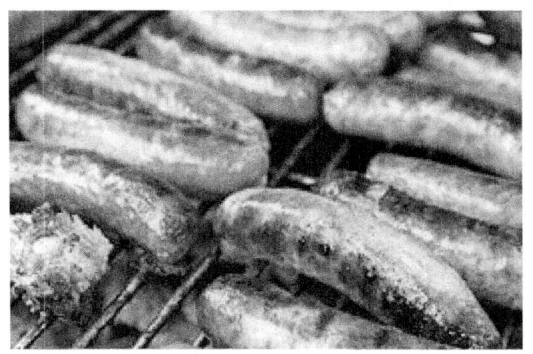

Pork Sausages

Total Prep and Cooking Time: 15 Minutes
Yields: 8 Servings
Nutrition Facts:
Calories: 138
Protein: 15 g
Net Carbs: 1 g
Fat: 8 g

Ingredients

1. 1 lb. ground pork
2. ½ tsp. kosher salt
3. ½ tsp. black pepper
4. ½ tsp. dried sage
5. ¼ tsp. allspice
6. 1/8 tsp. ground nutmeg
7. 1/8 tsp. onion powder
8. 1/8 tsp. cayenne pepper

9. 1/8 tsp. red pepper flakes

Instructions

1. In a mixing bowl, combine all ingredients and use hands to mix well.
2. Form the mixture into 8 patties.
3. Pan-fry the patties until brown on both sides (about 8-10 minutes).

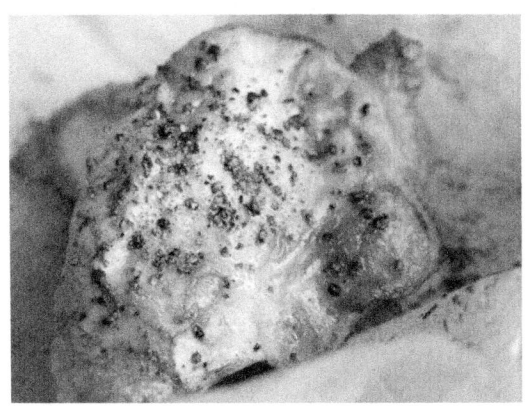

Simple Turkey Breast

Total Prep and Cooking Time: 1 hour 50 Minutes
Yields: 4 Servings
Nutrition Facts:
Calories: 385
Protein: 45 g
Net Carbs: 4.3 g
Fat: 11.8 g

Ingredients

1. 1 – 3 lb. turkey breast with skin on
2. ¼ cup soft butter
3. 1 clove of minced garlic
4. 1 tsp. paprika
5. 1 tsp. Italian seasoning
6. ½ tsp. garlic and herb seasoning
7. Salt and pepper to taste

8. 1 tbsp. butter
9. 1 cup chicken stock

Instructions

1. Mix the ¼ cup of butter with the paprika, garlic, Italian and herb seasonings.
2. Add in the salt and black pepper.
3. Place the turkey breasts with the skin side up in a roasting pan.
4. Make sure the skin is loose by slipping your fingers underneath and separating any connections.
5. Brush half of the butter mixture over the breasts (make sure your rub it underneath the skin).
6. Keep the remaining mixture for later.
7. Cover loosely with aluminum foil.
8. Pre-heat the oven to 350°F.
9. Roast the breasts for 1 hour.
10. Remove from oven and baste with the remaining butter mixture.
11. Return to oven and roast until the juices are clear.
12. Remove from oven and let rest for 15 minutes before serving.
13. Transfer drippings to a skillet.
14. Skim off the excess oil, reserving 1 tbsp.
15. Place skillet over a low fire.
16. Melt 1 tbsp. butter in the mixture.
17. Mix in the chicken stock.

18. Serve over the turkey breasts.

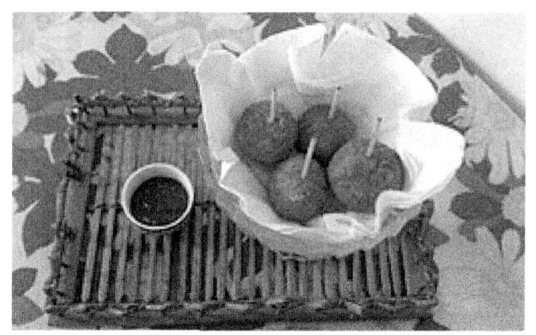

Carnivore Cheese Balls

Total Prep and Cooking Time: 30 Minutes
Yields: 8 Servings
Nutrition Facts:
Calories: 328
Protein: 12 g
Net Carbs: 3 g
Fat: 9 g

Ingredients

1. 1 cup shredded Cheddar cheese
2. 1 cup shredded Swiss cheese
3. 1 cup cream cheese
4. 2 tbsp. fresh chives
5. 2 tsp. Worcestershire sauce
6. ¼ tsp. smoked paprika
7. ½ tsp. garlic powder

Instructions

1. Place all the ingredients in a large mixing bowl.
2. Use your hands to mix them until well blended.
3. Shape the mixture into small balls and place them on a sheet of wax paper.
4. Refrigerate until time to serve.

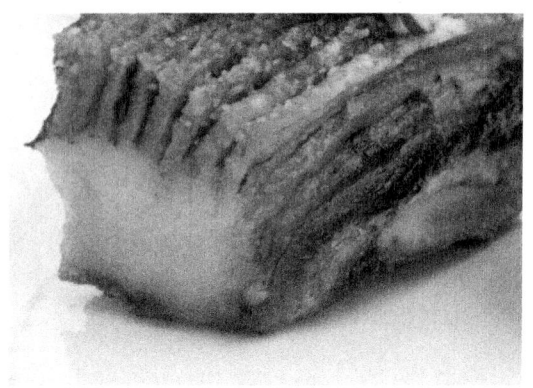

Pork Belly

Total Prep and Cooking Time: 1 hour 35 Minutes
Yields: 8 Servings
Nutrition Facts:
Calories: 297
Protein: 25 g
Net Carbs: 1 g
Fat: 30 g

Ingredients

1. 1 lb. slab of fresh pork belly
2. 2 tsp. fine salt
3. Pinch of black pepper

Instructions

1. Mix together the salt and black pepper into a dry rub.
2. Season the pork belly by rubbing it into the meat.
3. Cover and refrigerate overnight.
4. Preheat oven to 450°F.
5. Place pork belly into a roasting pan and cook in the oven for 30 minutes, fat side up.
6. Reduce heat to 275°F and roast for an additional hour or until tender.
7. Remove from oven and set aside to cool to room temperature.
8. Wrap in plastic wrap and refrigerate again until chilled all the way through.
9. Remove from refrigerator and slice into thick pieces.
10. Place in a frying pan and cook until nice and crispy.

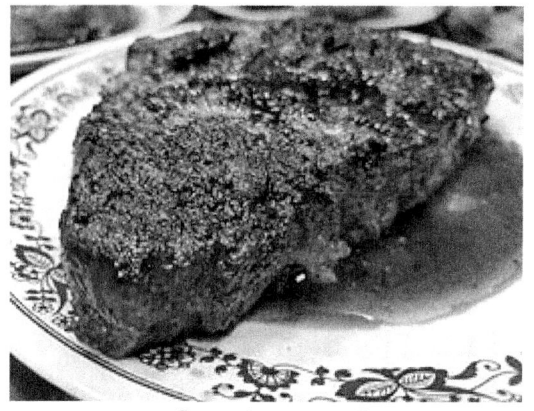

Classic Steak

Total Prep and Cooking Time: 20 Minutes
Yields: 4-6 Servings
Nutrition Facts: Calories: 479
Protein: 34 g
Net Carbs: 0 g
Fat: 8.5 g

Ingredients

1. 1 ½ lb. steaks

For the marinade:

1. 1/3 cup soy sauce
2. 3 tbsp. lime juice
3. 2 tbsp. balsamic vinegar

4. 3 tbsp. bacon fat + additional for the grill
5. 2 tbsp. parsley chopped fine
6. 1 tbsp. garlic minced
7. Kosher salt and black pepper to taste

Instructions

1. Score both sides of the steak with a sharp knife about ½" apart.
2. Blend together all of the ingredients in a large mixing bowl.
3. Pour marinade into a shallow glass dish or a Ziploc bag.
4. Place the scored steaks in the marinade and cover.
5. Let rest in the refrigerator for a minimum of 4 hours (maximum 8 hours).
6. Remove meat from marinade and let it stand for 30 minutes or until the meat is room temperature.
7. Use the bacon fat and preheat the pan.
8. Season steak with salt and pepper.
9. Cook in hot grease for about 3-4 minutes on each side or until you reach your desired level.
10. Remove from grill and let rest for 10 minutes before serving.

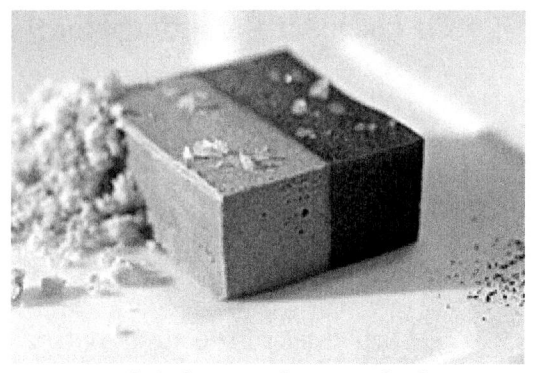

Chicken Liver Pâté

Total Prep and Cooking Time: 30 Minutes
Yields: 4 Servings
Nutrition Facts:
Calories: 539
Protein: 20 g
Net Carbs: 16 g
Fat: 43 g

Ingredients

1. 13 oz. of unsalted butter
2. 14 oz. chicken livers
3. 2 large cloves of garlic – 1 crushed and one sliced thin
4. 3 sprigs of thyme (leaves only)
   ¼ tsp. crushed cloves

Instructions

1. Heat up 1 tbsp of butter in a non-stick frying pan over medium heat.
2. Cook until the butter begins to foam.
3. Add in the chicken livers and fry for 2 minutes on both sides.
4. Stir in the crushed garlic and half of the thyme.
5. Fry for an additional 2 minutes.
6. Transfer the mixture to a food processor.
7. Blend into a smooth paste.
8. Season to taste.

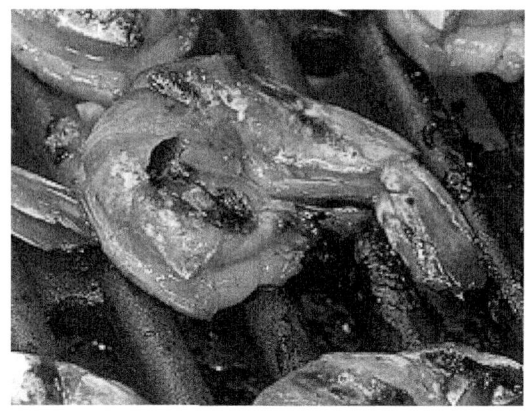

Grilled Shrimp

Total Prep and Cooking Time: 10 Minutes
Yields: 4 Servings
Nutrition Facts:
Calories: 102
Protein: 28 g
Net Carbs: 1 g
Fat: 3 g

Ingredients

For the shrimp seasoning:

1. 1 tsp. garlic powder
2. 1 tsp. kosher salt

3. ¼ tsp. cayenne pepper

For the shrimp:

1. 2 tbsp. bacon fat or lard
2. 1 tbsp. fresh lemon juice
3. 1 lb. jumbo shrimp peeled and de-veined

Instructions

1. Pre-heat a pan to a high temperature.
2. In a large mixing bowl, mix together the seasoning ingredients.
3. Drizzle in the bacon fat and lemon juice and stir until it becomes a paste.
4. Add the shrimp to bowl and toss to coat thoroughly.
5. Thread the shrimp onto metal skewers that have been soaked in water for an hour.
6. Brush the pan with bacon fat/lard.
7. Cook the shrimp until pink and opaque (about 2-3 minutes on each side).
8. Serve immediately.

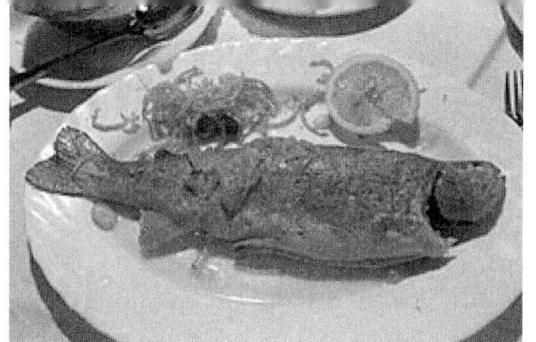

Poached Rainbow Trout

Total Prep & Cooking Time: 40 min.
Yields: 2 Servings
Nutrition Facts:
Calories: 218
Protein: 25 g
Net Carbs: 18 g
Fat: 6 g

Ingredients

1. 6 to 8 slices of lemon
2. 2 cups chicken broth
3. 2 boneless trout with skin on
4. Pinch of salt
5. Pinch of black pepper

Instructions

1. In a large skillet, place the lemon slices in a layer along the bottom.
2. Pour in the chicken broth.
3. Place over medium heat and bring the broth to a gentle simmer.
4. Season trout with salt and pepper.
5. Gently slide the trout over the lemons.
6. Cover and simmer for 8 minutes or until you see the flesh is opaque and flakes easily with a fork.
7. Remove from pan and place on a plate.
8. Spoon the lemon mixture over the trout and serve.

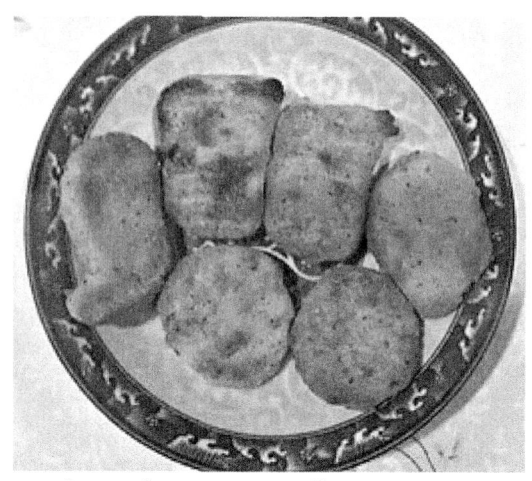

Carnivore Steak Nuggets

Total Prep & Cooking Time: 25 Minutes
Yields: 4 Servings
Nutrition Facts:
Calories: 609
Protein: 43 g
Net Carbs: 2 g
Fat: 38 g

Ingredients

1. 1 lb. venison or beef steak cut into chunks
2. 1 large egg
3. 1/2 oz. lard
4. ½ cup of grated parmesan cheese

5. ½ cup of pork panko
6. ½ tsp. of seasoned salt
7. ¼ cup mayonnaise
8. Juice from one medium lime

Instructions

For the breading

1. Mix together the pork panko, parmesan cheese, seasoned salt and set aside.

For the nuggets

1. In one bowl, beat the egg.
2. In a separate bowl, put in the breading mixture.
3. Dip the steak chunks in the egg mixture, then into the breading mixture.
4. Place breaded chunks on a sheet of wax paper.
5. Freeze chunks for 30 minutes to ensure that the breading will not fall off during frying.
6. In a large skillet, heat the lard to 325°F
7. Fry steak nuggets in batches until they have a nice golden brown color (about 2-3 minutes).
8. Transfer to a plate lined with paper towels.
9. Season with salt and serve.

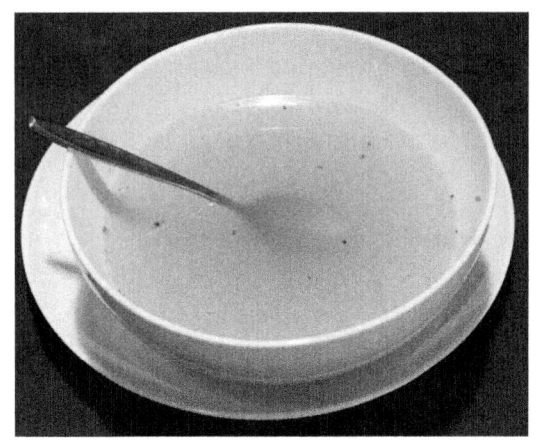

Beginner's Bone Broth

Total Prep and Cooking Time: 8+ hours
Yields: 16 Servings
Nutrition Facts:
Calories: 69
Protein: 6 g
Net Carbs: 1 g
Fat: 4 g

Ingredients

1. 4 lbs. mixed beef bones
2. 2 medium carrots
3. 3 celery stalks chopped
4. 2 medium onions chopped
5. 1 tbsp. melted lard

6. 2 tbsp. apple cider vinegar
7. 1 bay leaf

Instructions

1. Pre-heat oven to 400°F.
2. Place mixed bones in a large roasting pan coated with lard.
3. Roast bones in the oven for 30 minutes.
4. Turn over bones and roast for another 30 minutes.
5. Put roasted bones and all other ingredients in a stockpot.
6. Cover completely with water and bring to a simmer.
7. Lower the heat and allow it to simmer for another 8+ hours.
8. Continue to add water as needed (you want to kccp all the ingredients submerged).
9. The broth is done when it takes on a dark rich brown color.
10. Remove from heat and discard the bones and all other ingredients.
11. Strain the broth through a wire strainer or cheesecloth.
12. Allow it to cool down to room temperature.
13. Pour into jars and let it cool in the refrigerator.
14. When ready to eat, heat to your desired temperature before serving.

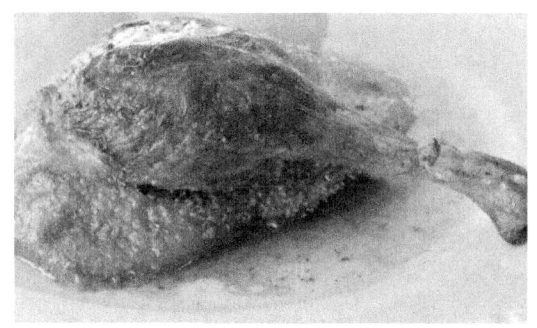

Duck Leg Confit

Total Prep and Cooking Time: 15 hours
Yields: 4 Servings
Nutrition Facts:
Calories: 223
Protein: 32 g
Net Carbs: 2.5 g
Fat: 25 g

Ingredients

1. 4 duck legs, excess fat trimmed and reserved
2. 1 tablespoon sea salt
3. 1/2 teaspoon freshly ground black pepper
4. 10 garlic cloves
5. 4 bay leaves
6. 4 sprigs fresh thyme

7. 1 1/2 teaspoons black peppercorns
8. 1/2 teaspoon table salt
9. 4 cups duck fat

Instructions

1. Lay the leg portions on a platter, skin-side down. Sprinkle with the sea salt and black pepper. Place the garlic cloves, bay leaves and sprigs of thyme on 2 leg portions. Lay the other 2 leg portions, flesh to flesh, on top. Cover and refrigerate for 12 hours.
2. Preheat the oven to 300°F.
3. Remove the duck from the refrigerator. Rinse with cool water, rubbing off some of the salt and pepper. Pat dry with paper towels.
4. Sprinkle peppercorns and salt evenly in a skillet. Lay the duck on top, skin-side down. Add the duck fat. Cover and bake for 2.5 to 3 hours, or until the meat pulls away from the bone.
5. Remove the duck from the fat.
6. To serve, sear duck legs skin-side down in a hot pan until the skin is golden and crispy.

Further Resources

Websites
www.zerocarbzen.com
www.zerocarbhealth.com
www.highsteaks.com
www.paleostyle.com
www.carnivorewiki.com
www.reddit.com/r/zerocarb

Facebook Groups
Zeroing In On Health
Zero Carb Health
World Carnivore Tribe
Principia Carnivora
Zero Carb UK

Twitter
@KetoCarnivore
@SBakerMD
@CarnivoresCreed
@GeorgiaEdeMD
@franktufan
@bendormiki
@MikhailaAleksis

YouTube Channels
Shawn Baker
Sv3rige
Mikhaila Peterson
KetOMAD

About the Author

Stephen Baker is a married father of two who lives in Branson, Missouri. He has been a health writer for over 20 years and his passions include mountain biking and crossfit.

Printed in Great Britain
by Amazon